DEPARTMENT · OF HEALTH ·

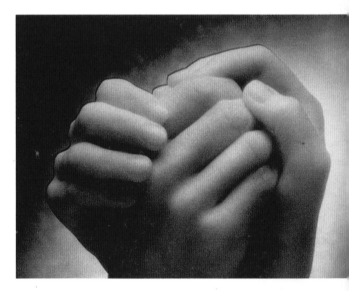

WORKING
IN PARTNERSHIP

A collaborative approach to care

REPORT OF THE

MENTAL HEALTH

NURSING REVIEW TEAM

610.7368   DEP

HMSO publications are available from:

HMSO Publications Centre
(Mail, fax and telephone orders only)
PO Box 276, London SW8 5DT
Telephone orders 071-873 9090
General enquiries 071-873 0011
(queuing system in operation for both numbers)
Fax orders 071-873 8200

HMSO Bookshops
49 High Holborn, London WC1V 6HB
071-873 0011 Fax 071-873 8200 (counter service only)
258 Broad Street, Birmingham B1 2HE
021-643 3740 Fax 021-643 6510
33 Wine Street, Bristol BS1 2BQ
0272 264306 Fax 0272 294515
9-21 Princess Street, Manchester M60 8AS
061-834 7201 Fax 061-833 0634
16 Arthur Street, Belfast BT1 4GD
0232 238451 Fax 0232 235401
71 Lothian Road, Edinburgh EH3 9AZ
031-228 4181 Fax 031-229 2734

HMSO's Accredited Agents
(see Yellow Pages)

and through good booksellers

Foreword

The last decade has seen dramatic changes in the way in which mental health services are organised and, indeed, changes in our whole approach to the concept of mental health itself. The NHS reforms and major recent policy initiatives – Caring for People, Health of the Nation, the Children Act and Patient's Charter – have proved to be major forces in driving forward change. Together, they are making a real and positive impact on the way that services are delivered, with an important and much needed shift in emphasis from secondary to primary care. Mental health nurses have a key role in ensuring that patients receive a high-quality service in this challenging new era.

The hallmark of a quality service is that it is sensitive and responsive to people's individual needs. This report rightly calls for a collaborative approach to meet that goal. It recognises that mental health nurses need to foster effective partnerships – between people who use services and their carers, between health professionals, across disciplines and between providers and commissioners of care.

Mental health nurses have a pivotal role to play in the health care team and they will need to be properly equipped with the skills to do so. They need the skills to care for people with acute and enduring mental illness. They need to be able to assess, plan, implement and evaluate care. Their profession needs to act both as practitioners and key workers in varied and diverse health care teams. Their work requires the ability to move confidently between hospital and community settings and to respond quickly and creatively to the rapidly changing demands of the service and its users.

I welcome this report as an excellent pointer to ways of ensuring that we have a well-qualified and motivated mental health nursing workforce. That is an essential part of any successful strategy for developing high quality services and for ensuring that patients receive the services that they need. With the skill, commitment and compassion that mental health nurses show in their working life, I am confident that they will rise to the challenges in the report.

Virginia Bottomley

Rt Hon Virginia Bottomley JP MP
Secretary of State for Health

Preface

To: *The Right Honourable Virginia Bottomley* JP MP

Secretary of State for Health

Dear Secretary of State

On behalf of the Mental Health Nursing Review Team I have the honour of submitting our report to you.

We have interpreted our terms of reference widely but the common theme running throughout our report concerns the profession's responsibilities to people who use mental health services.

We recommend that consultation with people who use services is built into the planning and development of all services, and that such consultation and partnership offers the prospect of major advances in mental health care. In our view, given the right support and encouragement, nurses will be in the vanguard of practice in the provision of mental health care.

The Review Team have identified how mental health nurses will take a central role in the provision of mental health services. Amongst our recommendations we urge that they focus their attention on people with serious and enduring mental illness including elderly people with mental illness, lead on acting as key workers and in systems of supervised discharge, and carry a central responsibility as providers of information to people who use services. We have identified exciting new roles involving advanced nursing practice in, for example, psychosocial intervention with people with schizophrenia and liaison nursing with accident and emergency services and general hospitals.

We ask for support to enable the development of high quality mental health nursing through the establishment of systems of clinical supervision, the provision of practice time for nurse educators and identifying the development needs of staff presently working in all residential care settings. Many of the nurses we spoke with question the therapeutic value of the District General Hospital psychiatric unit given the changing mix of the patient population. We also urge the provision of choice in single sex accommodation and gender of key worker and recommend attention to the provision of opportunities for partnerships with people who use services.

In order to meet these challenges it is essential that mental health nurses realise their full potential. They should be able to practise effectively and be accountable for the standards of care they provide. It is important that their education and training is not just appropriate for today's tasks, but that their education, their training and their experience will also equip them for the needs and tasks of tomorrow.

The key to any effective organisation is the quality and motivation of its staff, coupled with the need for positive leadership and an agreed agenda for action. This report, in our view, provides that impetus for change.

I would like to take this opportunity of thanking those who have contributed to the work of the review, especially the review team members for giving so generously of their time, energy and expertise to the review process; and my particular gratitude to John Archer, Geoff Bourne, Jean Faugier, Jo Lucas, Andrew McCulloch, and John Tait for unstinting support and advice as members of the Review Team's Editorial Board. Sincere thanks are due to our secretary Mr Clyde Lake, whose hard work, experience and diplomatic skills have been of the greatest value to our discussions and for ensuring continuity and coordination of our work. Our thanks are also due to the other members of the secretariat team, particularly Millie Carter and Frank Corr who have assisted Mr Lake and the Review Team in innumerable ways.

Professor Tony Butterworth

January 1994

Memberships

Professor Tony Butterworth, Chairman
Queen's Institute Professor of Community
Nursing, University of Manchester

Mr John Archer
Director of Nursing & Service Development
Community Priority Services
Tameside and Glossop Health Authority

Mrs Jean A Ball, Senior Teaching Fellow
Nuffield Institute for Health Studies
University of Leeds

Mrs Patricia Ball
Director of Clinical Services
The Mental Health Foundation
of Mid Staffordshire NHS Trust

Mr Geoff Bourne
Director, Mental Health and Learning Disability
Nursing, English National Board

Mr Martin Brown, Nursing Officer
Performance Management Directorate, NHSME

Mr Peter Campbell, Secretary
Survivors Speak Out

Mr Ian Cartwright
Director of Social Services, Doncaster

Mrs Edna Conlan, Chair
United Kingdom Advocacy Network

Professor Patrick Darcy
Director of Nurse Education Western Area
College of Nursing, Londonderry

Mr Philip Draper
Senior Clinical Nurse (Community)
United Bristol Healthcare NHS Trust

Dame Audrey Emerton
Formerly RNO
South East Thames RHA

Dr Ben Essex, General Practitioner
Sydenham Green Health Centre, London

Mrs Jean Faugier, Senior Lecturer in Nursing
University of Manchester

Miss Sonia Francis, SHANTI
Women's Counselling Project, London

Mr Sam Hetherington, Chief Executive
Avalon, Somerset NHS Trust

Dr Rachel Jenkins, Principal Medical Officer
Health Care Division, Department of Health

Mrs Hilary Kent
Formerly Regional Nursing Adviser
Northern RHA

Mr Seamus Killen
Formerly Director of Nursing Services
Littlemore Hospital, Oxford

Professor Israel Kolvin
Professor for Child & Family Mental Health
The Royal Free Hospital School of Medicine
and the Tavistock Centre, London

Ms Jo Lucas, Director of Development
National Association for Mental Health
(MIND)

Mr Steven Manikon
Nurse Advisor/Service Director
West Park Hospital, Surrey
(up to December 1993)

Mr Andrew McCulloch, Assistant Secretary
Health Care Division (Mental Health)
Department of Health

Ms Sue Ritter
Lecturer in Psychiatric Nursing
Institute of Psychiatry, London

Mrs Edna Robinson
Director of Community Care
Manchester DHAs Purchasing Consortium

Ms Lisa Rodrigues
Development Manager (Strategy)
South Downs Health NHS Trust

Mr Tom Sandford
Policy Adviser (Mental Health)
Royal College of Nursing, London

Mr Gareth Smith, Assistant Chief Inspector
Social Services Inspectorate (Mental Health)
Department of Health

Mr John Tait, Deputy Chief Nursing Officer
Department of Health

Mrs Sarah Waller, Head of Division
Personnel Development, NHSME

Terms of reference

To identify the future requirements for skilled nursing care in the light of developments in the provision of services for people with mental illness.

Contents

Executive summary

In April 1992, the Secretary of State for Health announced a new and comprehensive review of Mental Health Nursing. The last major review took place in 1968. The report from that review, *Psychiatric Nursing Today and Tomorrow* made a significant contribution to the development of Mental Health Nursing.

The current review explores the impact of changes in society and social policy since the late sixties, and their implications for practice, education, research and management in Mental Health Nursing.

We have interpreted our terms of reference widely but the common theme running throughout our report concerns the profession's responsibilities to people who use mental health services.

We took evidence from the broadest possible range of interested parties in mental health care. Consultative conferences, visits to clinical areas, written and oral evidence were all used to ensure comprehensive coverage of the issues. Our methods of working are described in detail in the early stages of the report.

Amongst our recommendations we urge that they focus their attention on people with serious and enduring mental illness including elderly people with mental illness, lead on acting as key workers and in systems of supervised discharge, and carry a central responsibility as providers of information to people who use services. We have identified exciting new roles involving advanced nursing practice, in for example, psychosocial intervention with people with schizophrenia and liaison nursing with accident and emergency services and general hospitals.

We reject the suggestion of the creation of a 'generic' nurse and the conversion of Mental Health Nursing to a post-registration specialty. We ask for support to enable the development of high quality Mental Health Nursing through the establishment of systems of clinical supervision, the provision of practice time for nurse educators and identifying the development needs of staff presently working in all residential care settings. Many of the nurses we spoke with question the therapeutic value of the District General Hospital Psychiatric Unit given the changing mix of the patient population. We also urge the provision of choice in single sex accommodation and gender of key worker and recommend attention to the provision of opportunities for partnerships with people who use services.

While collaboration and partnership with other disciplines are keys to successful mental health care, the core skills of the mental health nurse are reaffirmed and clarified. At the same time, clear protocols for the relative involvement of the various professions are essential.

We believe that the speed of change in society and social policy presents the Mental Health Nursing profession with exciting opportunities for new and enlightened developments in care. Nurses are already proving themselves to be effective and imaginative innovators in many areas of practice and we confidently anticipate a valuable – and valued – role for the mental health nurse in meeting the challenges of the future.

As approaches to care become increasingly centred on the individual, the mental health nurse's contribution – with its emphasis on interpersonal relationships and operational flexibility – will be critical to success.

The principle of choice for people who use services and their carers needs to be fully established as a basis for the practice of Mental Health Nursing.

The work of mental health nurses rests upon the relationship they have with people who use services. Our recommendations for future action start and finish with this relationship.

If we had to sum up our report in one recommendation, it would be that, "*Mental Health Nursing should re-examine every aspect of its policy and practice in the light of the needs of people who use services*". Nursing services should be designed and developed to meet the needs of people who use services: people should not be expected to conform to the convenience of the service.

Mental Health Nursing faces immense challenges in helping to meet the mental health needs of society. But we also believe that this is a period of great opportunity. Nurses need to foster a more constructive relationship with people who use services; they need to capitalise on their specialised skills to play a full part in the multidisciplinary team.

In rising to these challenges, mental health nurses will consolidate their position as key contributors to progressive, mental health services. This will bring greater professional rewards to the individual practitioner and, more importantly, it will bring major advances in the quality of care. Our vision for the future of mental health services places mental health nurses in the vanguard of practice: building on existing expertise and developing new skills; collaborating confidently and constructively with colleagues in the multidisciplinary team; and responding directly and appropriately to the needs of people who use services.

Introduction

The last official review of Mental Health Nursing *Psychiatric Nursing – Today and Tomorrow* took place in 1968.[1] The report focused particularly on in-patient psychiatric nursing. Since then there has been a fundamental shift in prevailing attitudes and philosophies of care, with a drive towards community-based services.

The Secretary of State's decision to establish a Review of Mental Health Nursing has met with widespread support from people who use services, their carers and voluntary bodies, as well as statutory and professional organisations.[2] The review is timely as there is a need to reflect on developments since 1968: these include changes in the legal framework, shifts in social, political and economic policy, alterations in public attitudes and expectations, and the move towards more individualised approaches to care.

This review of Mental Health Nursing provides an opportunity to respond to questions being raised by service providers, researchers and the profession at large. Debates have taken place on the focus of work for mental health nurses in the reprovision of services particularly those working in the community.[3] [4] Predications have also been made about the future direction of the profession[5] and a detailed report of Mental Health Nursing has been undertaken by the Royal College of Nursing and submitted as evidence.

Mental Health Nursing practice must change and develop to meet the challenges of clients' needs in all their different circumstances. It is important to recognise that although Mental Health Nursing is concerned with the individual, it operates within multi-disciplinary teams within a multi-agency service. In order to provide a comprehensive range of user-orientated services in which Mental Health Nursing can play its part, close collaboration is essential; this will include the agreement of a common strategy between participating health services, local authority services and non-statutory agencies.

Mental health nurses have a key role to play in the future development of high-quality mental health services. It is vital that they are properly prepared as practitioners to meet the needs of clients. The Review Team have drawn substantially on information gained from a wide-ranging consultation exercise conducted in the first phase of the review. Consequently this report is informed by the views of people who use services, their carers, professionals, commissioners, providers, and both statutory and non-statutory agencies.

This report provides a vision of how best to equip and deploy valuable Mental Health Nursing resources to best effect. It sets out the future role and function of mental health nurses, and their potential contribution in a wide variety of settings – as individual practitioners, or as members of multi-disciplinary and multi-agency care teams. It also provides a framework for action which takes account of policy developments, organisational changes and educational requirements in order to meet the changing needs of people for whom services are provided.

"... the widest possible consultation

1.0 THE BACKGROUND

and input into the review process..."

1.1

Methods of working

In view of the complexity of the issues involved, the Review Team decided to divide into five specialised sub-groups covering the following areas of study: consumer affairs; education; practice; research; and structural issues. It was also agreed that co-opted members would be invited to join the working groups to maximise the groups' effectiveness. Wherever possible, the groups met on the same day in order to facilitate the exchange of information.

The Review Team were anxious to ensure the widest possible consultation and input into the review process and agreed that evidence would be obtained from written and oral sources, regional conferences and visits to clinical practice areas. Written evidence was invited from Regional Health Authorities, District Health Authorities, Family Health Service Authorities, NHS Trusts (Mental Health), Social Services Departments, Community Health Councils, Special Health Authorities, professional and statutory bodies, individual practitioners, people who use services and their carers, and other relevant agencies in the public, private and voluntary sectors (Annex A).

Three regional consultative conferences were held which brought users, carers, professionals, statutory bodies and voluntary agencies together with members of the Review Team (Annex B).

Oral evidence was taken from individuals, organisations and groups representing a wide range of specialist expertise (Annex C).

We undertook a number of visits. The locations provided a wide geographical perspective around the country and included services in inner city, urban and rural areas. The visits encompassed a large spectrum of service types, including acute adult services in a district general hospital; community services; ethnic services; services for homeless people; child and adolescent mental health services; crisis intervention services; services for elderly people; rehabilitation; interchange with general hospital services, especially Accident and Emergency; liaison psychiatry; specialist services; and drop-in centres (Annex D).

The Review Team have drawn heavily on the responses received from all sources, including written evidence, oral contributions, conference transcripts, clinical visit data and the work of the sub-groups. We gratefully acknowledge the interest, work and support of the many people who contributed to these activities.

The context

The starting point

This review starts from a belief that the work of mental health nurses rests on their relationship with people who use mental health services. This relationship should have value to both partners. It is important that the recommendations of the review are more than rhetoric or fashionable statements of ideology. We have attempted to address matters in this review in such a way that the final product is of positive value to people who use services, mental health nurses and other professional groups.

The settings for practice

In the 25 years since the last report on Mental Health Nursing,[1] there have been significant changes in service provision, professional roles, research, education and – most importantly of all – the expression given to the interests of service-users. It is therefore impossible to consider Mental Health Nursing without taking account of the settings in which it is practised.

People who use services

We wish to emphasise the positive effect that nursing can have on the lives of people who use services. It is acknowledged that Mental Health Nursing has not always been successful in providing good quality services which respond to people in their care. The review recognises the impact of the 'compulsory' nature of the relationship between nurses and some service-users. The principle of user and carer choice needs to be firmly established as a basis for the practice of Mental Health Nursing.

The role of mental health nurses

The numerous demands of policy change which surrounded this review added to doubts about the role of mental health nurses – perhaps an inevitable consequence of a period which has seen such dramatic change. The reprovision of services in the community, the re-organisation of nurse education, the demands for change from the greater profession of nursing and the evolving expectations of people who use services, have all combined to produce anxiety and uncertainty about the future role of Mental Health Nursing.

This review was conducted during a period when a number of forces were presenting new challenges to professional mental health nurses. We have had to rise to these challenges and be ready for radical proposals for change. We were prepared to consider the creation of a new type of mental health care worker, but in the event received little evidence to support such a development. We are convinced that the mental health nurse should play a central role in the provision of high-quality mental health care.

1.2.5 Developing a partnership

Developing partnerships with people who use services carries complex and subtle demands. To encourage such development, nurses have to appreciate and be honest about the limitations of mental health services and the uncertainty of solutions; they should respond to people's expressed needs, taking them seriously and, wherever possible, providing choice. People who use services should be given real choice in matters of care. Choice should be offered in areas such as the gender of the named nurse, types of treatment and the practicalities of daily living.

1.2.6 Working within policy for the provision of mental health services

Mental Health Nursing should be understood within a background of wider changes in the NHS, including – most importantly – the commissioning/provider system which has proved to be a major force in driving forward change in a number of key policy areas. This, together with *The NHS and Community Care Act* 1990,[6] *The Children Act* 1989,[7] *The Patient's Charter*[8] and *Health of the Nation*,[9] is having a significant impact on service delivery. The sum total of these policy initiatives provides an exciting and challenging new era for mental health. Mental health nurses have a key role in ensuring that these policies work effectively and help to deliver a high-quality service.

1.2.7 The education of mental health nurses

Despite clear evidence of innovative and exciting career opportunities, research indicates a progressive fall in recruitment to Mental Health Nursing courses in the last decade (Annex E). It has also been suggested that the subject of Mental Health Nursing is being compromised by its generic alignment in Project 2000 nurse education programmes, and concern has also been expressed about the quality of continuing education for qualified mental health nurses.

1.2.8 Multi-disciplinary and multi-agency working

The significant development of multi-agency and multi-disciplinary working raises questions about issues of power and control over resources. This review begins from an understanding that, while financial accountability remains with a responsible authority, there should be shared responsibility for development of services, based on the needs of users rather than the priorities of agencies or professional groups. Boundaries established to safeguard professional integrity should not prevent work in different settings. Rather they should provide a framework to support the unique role, value and skills of mental health nurses, and the other professions involved.

"We are convinced that the mental health nurse

2.0 THE ISSUES

should play a central role in the provision of

high-quality mental health care in a range of settings"

Expectations of mental health nurses

It is a fundamental right that, *"people who use mental health services can expect to receive skilled, sensitive, professional support from competent mental health nurses."*

2.1.1

Issues in context

There have been significant failures in the past which should not be forgotten or ignored. Abuse and neglect of the most vulnerable people in our care have been widely reported in a series of inquiries – and they are as distressing to mental health nurses as they are to the population at large. Invariably the evidence in these cases points to inappropriate attitudes of staff, poor management of services and insufficient support or continuing education for staff, often exacerbated by ineffective or absent quality control measures.

Recommendations from these inquiries continue to be relevant and are supported by the Review Team. The problems reported are a consequence of deficiencies in the delivery of mental health services as a whole and are not necessarily specific to nurses. Nonetheless, nurses can make a significant contribution to their eradication.

Recent research has shown that people who have been in psychiatric hospitals value the nursing care they receive.[11] 59% of respondents to the survey said that they were either satisfied or very satisfied with nursing care. While this indicates some satisfaction with mental health nurses in hospitals, the views of those who did not respond positively need our particular attention.

2.1.2

Identifying discrimination

MIND's *Stress on Women* campaign presented evidence that abuse of women is startlingly common within mental health services.[12] [13] This is particularly worrying given the growing recognition that many women who are admitted to psychiatric hospital are victims of childhood sexual abuse. We return to this issue in Section 2.4.

The Review Team also heard that people from black and other minority ethnic groups are consistently treated differently within the psychiatric system. Young Afro-Caribbean men are more likely to be admitted compulsorily under the Mental Health Act 1983 – and treated with less understanding when they are in hospital.[14] Research shows that Irish people have similar experiences.[15] People from Asian and some other ethnic minority groups are significantly under-represented within the services. Services that are designed specifically for these latter groups get a very good take-up, so it is clear that the problem is with access to mainstream services, and not because of a low morbidity rate or because communities prefer to rely on their own resources.[16]

Nurses should meet racial and culture-specific needs, if necessary by finding novel and creative solutions to practical problems. Staff from black and ethnic minority groups can have a valuable part to play, but their involvement should not be a substitute for universal training in the needs of minority groups. Managers should ensure that their services are sensitive to the needs of local black and ethnic minority populations. This includes recruiting staff that reflect the local community, providing access to interpreters and ensuring that dietary needs are met. It will require specific recruitment and training programmes – and consultation with local community groups.

Recommendation 1
We recommend that nurses improve their understanding and awareness of the racial and cultural needs of people who use services and ensure that these are fully reflected when developing care plans.

2.1.3

Information

We heard that requests for information from people using services were met with varying degrees of courtesy and helpfulness. Mental health nurses can play a central role in making sure that not only are people's minimum legal rights to information honoured, but that they also have access to the full range of information about local services and treatment options as well as the effects of medication. Where appropriate, people should also be informed about their rights of access to their own clinical notes.

People who use services report that informed consent is not always implemented in frequently-used treatments such as phenothiazines. This raises concerns that some nurses are involved in poor practice by ignoring their responsibilities for protecting the rights of the people in their care. The relative absence of discussion on these issues in the professional press, educational curricula or research provides further worrying indicators.

The needs of carers are often ignored. Carers need information about the care provided, possible treatment options, the effects of medication and the likely outcomes. However, mental health nurses have to be aware that some people who use services will not want their carers to be directly involved in their care plan. They should respect this wish and support them in maintaining it, whilst giving the appropriate information to carers. In some circumstances, nurses need support in managing the conflicts of interest that can arise. It is also very important to recognise that the person identified as the carer may not be the nearest relative.

Nurses should give people accurate information about their rights in a way which it is easy for an individual to consider, understand and act upon. 'Telling people things' is not enough. Managers should ensure that information resources are available and translated into the language of the local community where necessary.

Recommendation 2
We recommend that mental health nurses take a lead role in ensuring that people in their care have access to appropriate information, including treatment options and rights.

A practical innovation

2.1.4

The Review Team heard evidence from people who, during a crisis admission to hospital, had been unable to convince staff of the validity of their concerns about particular drugs or therapies. The use of innovative 'crisis cards', now supported by many user groups, is being adopted by some services. This system is similar to those used by people with diabetes or allergies to medication: it identifies the most effective response in cases of crisis and the people who should be involved. They can be particularly important in identifying adverse reactions to specific medication.

Recommendation 3
We recommend that managers introduce a system of holding and acting upon information about people's wishes and needs in crisis.

2.1.5   **Challenging behaviour and personal dignity**

The issue of personal dignity was a recurring theme in evidence to the review. Nurses have to deal with difficult and sometimes threatening situations, but there are ways to deal with such situations (including those requiring restraint) in such a way as to preserve the dignity of the individual. It was recognised that maintaining dignity requires adequate levels of suitably trained staff. We heard evidence from a number of groups and individuals who were concerned that staffing levels and/or skill mix were in some cases inappropriate.

The use of seclusion was also raised in evidence by many of the people who use services. We believe that where seclusion is still used, it should be carefully monitored and not used as an automatic response to challenging behaviour. Alternative responses to aggressive or disturbed behaviour should always be considered. We return to these issues in Section 2.4.

2.1.6   **Relationships**

Recent National Health Service policies recognise the importance of people who use services. Many of the changes specify consultation with carers and the involvement of individuals in their own treatment. It follows that the future of Mental Health Nursing, whether based in the community, residential or hospital settings, should focus on the quality of the relationship between the nurse, the person using services and any 'significant others', be they family, friends or partners.

The implementation of these policies requires a different way of working with users and carers, based on a relationship of understanding and respect. A good way to start is to involve users and carers as trainers on professional training courses. There is a growing number of people who have used services who have the skills and experience to take part in professional training. The national networks also have contacts with skilled user trainers across the country.

People who use services also have an important role to play in advising commissioners and informing the process of mental health needs assessment. This valuable contribution should be harnessed by ensuring that local user groups are represented on the Boards of Commissioning Agencies – as is happening in some areas already.

Recommendation 4
We recommend the representation and participation of people who use services on service planning, education and research groups.

2.1.7   **The question of advocacy**

National user groups are applying some of their resources to help local support groups who want to become involved with advocacy, local planning, service management, teaching or research. A substantial number of action and support groups now offer help and advocacy, enabling individuals and groups to be more articulate in expressing their views and achieving positive change. They also support individuals and groups in the delivery of training and consultancy to the statutory services.

Unfortunately, nurses still face difficulties in speaking out on behalf of those most vulnerable to the negative effects of poor service provision. Users report there is a tendency for some professionals to close ranks rather than confront bad practice. This cannot be condoned.

At the same time, there have been some excellent developments in which nurses have spoken out on behalf of their clients, often at some risk to their own positions. The Review Team are clear, however, that mental health nurses cannot be independent advocates. Because they are part of the service, there is a potential conflict of interest with their role as employees, their duty of care and their professional ethics. Nurses should speak out on behalf of the people in their care, but service-users should also have access to advocates on the wards or in the community, who can express their wishes and views unreservedly.

Mental health nurses have a critical role in ensuring that the people in their care know about advocacy services and that advocates are welcomed and listened to. Mental health nurses also have an important role in ensuring that the wishes and needs of people who are very disabled by their mental health problems are acknowledged. This group of people may not be very articulate and it is important that their voice is not lost.

Whilst it is essential to specify the need for an honest and open relationship, this honesty should be balanced by the recognition that nurses (and other mental health professionals) have the power to detain people and compel them to take part in treatment against their will. In exerting this authority, mental health nurses have to be skilled and sensitive if they are to earn the confidence of people in this unequal relationship.

Individual responsibility

2.1.8

Mental health nurses are accountable to people who use services, the organisation within which they work and to their statutory professional organisations.

Accountability begins with an appreciation of the nurse's own potential and value as a human being, and a recognition of his or her own limitations. Accountability brings the potentially uncomfortable responsibility of speaking out against bad practice, including those measures which militate against the freedom and choice of the individual. Failure to do so damages the trust which is so critical to the therapeutic relationship. Accountability should be seen as a liberating influence rather than a constraint. However, if nurses are to exercise individual accountability, they should have a clear idea of what is expected from them, especially in the more challenging and difficult areas of practice.

Nurses should also be aware of the implications of the Patient's Charter and any local mission statements and policies which set standards for practice. Managers should ensure the necessary staffing levels and skill mix to support good practice and facilitate professional accountability. They should also help to create a culture where staff feel confident to speak out against abuses in the system.

The review noted with concern the disproportionate numbers of disciplinary cases brought to the UKCC which involve male mental health nurses and female patients.

Recommendation 5
We recommend that the UKCC investigates and reports on the disproportionate numbers of disciplinary cases which involve male nurses and female patients.

2.2

The practice of mental health nurses

We are convinced that mental health nurses should play a central role in the provision of high-quality mental health care in a range of settings, but the scope of their involvement should be clearly defined. Given the high morbidity of mental health problems in the community, the demand for services cannot be met by mental health nurses alone, it requires a strong partnership both with and within the Primary Health Care Team (*see page 27 – Particular requirement of the Primary Health Care Team*).

This review generated considerable debate about a 'proper' focus for the work of mental health nurses. In response to the high potential morbidity in primary health care, nurses have made a significant contribution by adjusting their practice, developing their role to accept direct referrals and providing outreach services. However, one consequence of this has been a shift in focus away from people with more severe problems, such as schizophrenia. Eighty per cent of people with schizophrenia in England have not been on the caseload of a mental health nurse working in the community.[17] This suggests that strategic decisions made by service managers and individual mental health nurses have not always targeted the people in greatest need.

Recommendation 6
We recommend that the essential focus for the work of mental health nurses lies in working with people with serious or enduring mental illness in secondary and tertiary care, regardless of setting.

2.2.1

Affirming the role of the mental health nurse

We are aware that some people have expected this review to recommend the creation of a 'generic' nurse and the conversion of Mental Health Nursing to a post-registration speciality, others have cautioned against this view.[18] In fact, we do not favour this approach and have seen little evidence of support for such an idea. In our view, the 'generic' preparation of social work in the UK has not been a success for psychiatry and should not be repeated by nursing. Mental Health Nursing should be retained as a specialist qualification at initial level and *developed* at advanced levels.

Recommendation 7
We recommend that Mental Health Nursing should retain its specialty at initial preparation level.

The series of cases which involved such appalling mistreatment of residents in long-stay mental hospitals has cast a shadow over all the professions involved, including Mental Health Nursing. However, the Review Team would like to emphasise the excellent record of innovation and good practice of the profession at large. Indeed, on many occasions in recent times it has been nurses who have led service developments in opposition to more traditional views. Examples of this can be seen in a variety of nurse therapies, outreach services, liaison mental health nursing and a number of innovative schemes within the criminal justice system.

Skills of the mental health nurse

It is important to re-affirm the core skills of the mental health nurse. A pamphlet published by the Department of Health, 'Mental Illness: What does it mean?' has identified the common contribution of the mental health care team as a whole but there are very specific core skills which define and distinguish the contribution of Mental Health Nursing.[19] It suggests that in common:–

"Doctors, psychologists, nurses, social workers and occupational therapists work as mental health teams in most areas. They have some skills in common, such as counselling, and some that are particular to their individual training."

and that in particular:–

"Nursing staff are the largest group of trained staff dealing with people with mental health problems. They work in residential settings, including psychiatric units and nursing homes and as community psychiatric nurses. Their training equips them with counselling as well as caring, rehabilitation and medication supervision skills".

The skills of Mental Health Nursing have been clearly articulated by the English National Board under the headings of *Assessment, Planning, Implementation and Evaluation* (Annex F).

It is difficult to lay any exclusive claim to the possession of these skills, as other professional groups also operate from related knowledge and skills bases. However it is the combination of these particular skills, together with the values and practice common to the nursing profession as a whole, which provides the unique expertise of mental health nurses enabling them to:

- *establish a therapeutic relationship which rests in a respect for others and skilled therapeutic use of self*

- *sustain such relationships over time and respond flexibly to the changing needs of those with mental health problems*

- *construct, implement and evaluate a care programme*

- *provide skilled assessment, ongoing monitoring*

- *make risk assessments and judgements*

- *monitor the dosage, effects and contra indications of medication*

- *detect early signs of deteriorating mental health including potential self harm and suicide risk, worsening physical conditions and potential threats to others*

- *prioritise work in order to respond to those most in need*

- *collaborate with all members of the multi-disciplinary team*

- *network effectively, setting appropriate boundaries to professional input*

- *manage the therapeutic environment, determined by a clear awareness of issues such as safety, dignity, partnership.*

The experience of mental ill health is an individual one and inherently variable. In responding to the variety of mental health problems, Mental Health Nursing draws on a range of core skills that are grounded in the therapeutic use of self within the central relationship with the client.

The uniqueness of nursing is not essentially concerned with definitions which centre on professional prerogative: it should be based on a client-centred philosophy, the synthesis of knowledge upon which it draws, and, most importantly, its flexibility and responsiveness to individual needs.

2.2.3

The primacy of the individual

Nursing responses and interventions should be founded upon a sound understanding of the individuals in their care. Nurses need to treat all people who use services as equal partners and stake-holders in the service, recognising that they are people first – and 'clients' second.

Care begins with a formal and thorough assessment of needs, involving people who use services and their carers. At the same time, nurses need to collaborate openly and fully with others involved in mental health care – including other professionals, people from the voluntary sector and partners or 'significant others'.

The wishes of people who use services should be incorporated into every care plan and special note be made if they have been overridden by the duty of care. When planning care, nurses must be aware of the options for intervention – and their implications and likely outcomes. The nurse will also need to negotiate care packages with each person in their care, being open and explicit about the risks and implications of different strategies.

When implementing care, nurses are responsible for working within the bounds of their individual competence. The effects of nursing intervention should be systematically monitored from the first meeting with the client through to the termination of the contract. To help in this process, nurses should keep clear, contemporaneous and accurate records of care.[20]

Nurses need to acknowledge the current stigma of mental illness and its social effects on everybody involved. They should take every opportunity to combat stigma, wherever it exists.

Recommendation 8
We recommend that care plans should be developed with individuals and based on their wishes and needs – not the convenience of the service.

Nurses should spend time with people in their care in a way that makes sense to the individual and reflects his or her special needs. Doing this demands good listening skills and a commitment to understanding people, their background and the way they feel about their circumstances.

Managers should review staffing levels and working practices, and – if necessary – restructure them to enable nurses to spend more time with people in their care.

The Patient's Charter states that there should be a named registered nurse for each patient responsible for their nursing care. The advantages of the 'named nurse' system have recently been recognised in the programme of the Chief Nursing Officer, Department of Health: '*A Vision for the Future*'.[21] It states that "*...patient's new rights will influence not only the way in which the nursing profession provide services but also provide the opportunity for the profession to shape the way these standards are achieved. One example will be that mental health nurses and others will wish to take a positive approach not only to respecting patients' religious and cultural beliefs but the effect that these have on illness and behaviour...*"

Recommendation 9
We recommend that Mental Health Nursing services should be arranged to ensure that nurses spend the majority of their time responding to the needs of people who use services.

Approaches to practice   2.2.4

The Review Team found some evidence of practice which laid more emphasis on the task to be done, rather than a focus on the needs of the individual. It was clear that many services and individual nurses have introduced systematic individualised care plans and records of care, but their real impact on client care has yet to be fully evaluated.

Some practitioners who gave evidence struggled with the task of defining Mental Health Nursing and took a somewhat profession-specific rather than user-focused perspective. Their uncertainty may well have been precipitated by the speed of recent changes and the sense that services are still in a state of flux. The need to form alliances with people who use services has been highlighted by a wide range of fundamental policy initiatives, including *Working for Patients* (1989),[22] *The NHS & Community Care Act* (1990) and *The Patient's Charter* (1991). The Review Team wish to emphasise the importance of person-centred definitions of Mental Health Nursing.

During the course of the review, we have been provided with models of good Mental Health Nursing which demonstrate practice we wish to commend. Typically, these models include:

- a clearly informed assessment of client needs, which involves the clients and their carers

- an understanding of the needs and perceptions of the local community and positive efforts to promote awareness

- a conscious effort to deal sensitively with issues of race, creed and gender

- full and open collaboration with others, including colleagues from other professions, other nurses, midwives and health visitors and non-professional helpers

- accessibility and flexibility of managers

- identification of very clear objectives for intervention, clear measures of outcome and means of performance review

- the provision of high-quality managerial support for the mental health nurse, together with constant access to clinical supervision and continued professional development.

Mental Health Nursing is now being expressed at advanced practitioner level in such matters as psychosocial intervention with people with schizophrenia,[23] liaison mental health nursing in Accident & Emergency departments and court diversion schemes.

In addition to the core skills, mental health nurses can develop specialist skills appropriate to meeting specific needs of people in their care. Examples include counselling, family therapy, behaviour therapy, cognitive therapy and psychotherapy. However, these should complement rather than replace the core skills of the mental health nurse.

2.2.5   What's in a name?

All mental health nurses should be using the same core skills, irrespective of the setting within which they practice. Some nurses working within in-patient settings feel that their skills are undervalued, especially when compared to the often warm public acknowledgment of their colleagues working in the community. These views were particularly strong in units which served deprived inner-city areas, where nurses face unique challenges in providing appropriate care in demanding environments. The Review Team do not endorse such views: indeed the task of mental health nurses in residential and in-patient settings has particular challenges not experienced elsewhere in mental health care.

The Review Team appreciate and recognise the importance of the historic development of community psychiatric nursing services – and the part they have played in developing the profession and changing services. Nonetheless we believe that the continued separation between community and in-patient nursing militates against continuity of care. We recognise that there will continue to be mental health nurses who work exclusively in the community, but we suggest avoidance of terminology which discriminates between nurses working in community and in-patient settings.

Recommendation 10
We recommend that the title 'mental health nurse' be used both for nurses who work in the community and those who work in hospital and day services.

2.2.6   Clinical supervision

Recent reports have identified clinical supervision as an important development target for all nursing services. However, although the concept of clinical supervision is well accepted in Mental Health Nursing, it became apparent to us during the review that adequate clinical supervision is certainly not yet the norm for the majority of mental health nurses. For the most part, the only form of clinical supervision to which nurses have access is provided informally by their peer group.

There are notable exceptions, where there has been a sincere attempt to take the issue of clinical leadership and supervision seriously most commonly expressed through the role of advanced practitioner. However, such examples are few and far between. Even in those cases where attempts have been made to implement a cascade model of clinical supervision, it has often failed to include clinical managers, vital players in its provision. Nonetheless, from the examples of clinical supervision seen, together with emerging literature and policy recommendations, the importance of clinical supervision to Mental Health Nursing is clear.

Clinical supervision can take various guises, depending on the philosophy and style of the intervention being offered, but it is underpinned by a number of fundamental principles or ground rules (*Figure 1*).[24]

Figure I
Ground Rules for Clinical Supervision

- **Skills should be constantly re-defined and sophisticated throughout professional life**

- **Critical discussion about clinical practice is a means to professional development**

- **Introduction to the process of clinical supervision should begin in professional training and continue thereafter as an integral aspect of professional development**

- **Clinical supervision requires time, energy and commitment; it is not an incidental activity and must be planned and effectively resourced**

High-quality clinical supervision has many advantages:

- it places emphasis on clinical aspects of Mental Health Nursing

- it helps mental health nurses to assess training and research needs

- it encourages the recognition and appreciation of individual clients and their social situation

- it examines the multi-disciplinary contribution to comprehensive client care

- it identifies and develops innovative practice

- it creates an ethos which fosters staff retention and morale

- it promotes vital links between research and clinical practice.

There are three distinct but interrelated aspects of clinical supervision.[25] The *formative* or educational function aims to develop the skills, abilities and understanding of those supervised, by means of reflection and exploration.

The *restorative* or supportive function acknowledges that the 'therapeutic use of self' means just what it says: nurses will, of necessity, be affected by the pain and distress which is suffered by clients. The growth of primary nursing will inevitably increase this stress, and the need for clinical supervision.

Even those with most experience will have inevitable blind spots, human failings, areas of vulnerability and prejudices, of which they may remain unaware. The *normative* or managerial function of supervision supplies external quality control: it is up to the supervisor to ensure that the highest professional standards of nursing are upheld.

There is no doubt that if mental health nurses are to meet the challenges of the future, they should have access to skilled clinical supervision. Centrally funded initiatives are required to facilitate the implementation of clinical supervision, and managers may well need to restructure services to make it a reality.

Recommendation 11
We recommend that clinical supervision is established as an integral part of practice up to and including the level of advanced practitioner for mental health nurses.

2.2.7   **Difficult areas of clinical practice which should be governed by locally agreed policies**

The Review Team acknowledge the special demands placed on mental health nurses who manage often difficult clinical situations and though we have seen some very good practice certain issues were referred repeatedly to the Review Team for specific consideration.

These were:

Medication

The control of behaviour by medication requires careful thought. Medication which begins as a purely therapeutic intervention may, by prolonged routine administration, become a method of restraint. It is therefore necessary to review each case regularly. Medication should never be used as an alternative to adequate staffing or skill mix levels. It is also essential that nurses involved are fully conversant with the aims, possible side effects and contra-indications of each prescription they administer.

Time out

Time out is a behaviour modification technique which temporarily denies a person opportunity to participate in an activity or to receive positive reinforcers. It should be emphasised that this technique is used only as part of a planned behavioural modification and treatment programme. It should be seen as one of a range of planned methods of managing difficult behaviour; it should not be confused with seclusion.

Record keeping

It is important that appropriate, accurate and contemporaneous records of care and treatment are maintained.

The following practices should only be considered either as a last resort or when other strategies for care prove unsuitable. Aspects of these matters have been dealt with in detail in the Revised Code of Practice (1993) which was published during the course of this review.[26] The good practices outlined in that code have the full support of the Review Team and we would like to emphasise the importance of mental health nurses – and other health care workers – having a detailed working knowledge of both the Mental Health Act 1983[27] and its Code of Practice.

Locked doors

Mental health nurses are responsible for the care and protection of patients and staff and the maintenance of a safe environment. It may occasionally be necessary for the nurse in charge of a ward to lock the door of a ward (because of the behaviour of a patient or patients) to keep the environment safe. However, these occasions should be governed by a clearly articulated local policy.

Restraint

The purpose of restraint is firstly to take immediate control of a dangerous situation, and secondly to end or reduce significantly the threat to the individual involved or other people. Restraint limits the person's freedom and should be used for as short a time as possible and with respect to the individual's dignity.

Seclusion

Seclusion is the supervised confinement of an individual alone in a room, which may be locked to protect others from significant harm. It should be used as little as possible and for the shortest possible time. Many centres have now discontinued using seclusion altogether and the Review Team see this as a positive move.

Use of any of the above must be indicated by clinical need and governed by clearly articulated local policies.

2.3

Mental health nurses and service delivery

2.3.1

Management and leadership

Evidence presented to the Review Team showed no consensus on how nurses and nursing should be managed. Some believed that nurses can only be managed by clinically credible nurses, who would promote supervision and staff development. Such managers would provide professional leadership and achieve their career aspirations without having to enter general management positions. This view emphasised the value of a motivated, well trained and skilled workforce.

Many people expressed dismay at the lack of pro-active leaders who could grasp the opportunities of a developing service and take the lead in community developments. The contraction of long-stay hospitals had frequently resulted in the inappropriate transposition of hospital-based nurse management systems into the community, with no coherent strategy to sustain the new community orientation. Some respondents were critical of the quality of nurse managers, while others felt the major problem was the tendency for mental health to be seen as a low-priority area in comparison to other demands.

Usually there was a recognition that, since Mental Health Nursing was integrated with the work of other mental health professions and – indeed – many tasks overlapped considerably, the management of nurses could not be seen as the sole prerogative of nurses. This was felt to be reinforced by the increase in multi-agency partnerships and user-centred services.

General management is now the established model of health service management and mental health nurses need to recognise how their experience, training and education can equip them for a role within this system. In addition, mental health nurses are recognised to be particularly proficient in the area of people skills – expertise that is as essential to management as it is to clinical activity.

There was a firm belief that general management and leadership skills should be incorporated in nurse training from the beginning so that nursing qualifications could be seen as a firm basis for management development. Management, like education and research, should be integral to the activities of all trained nurses. Whilst there was a broad acceptance of general management, specific areas such as clinical standards, fitness to practise and other professional issues were seen as the legitimate concerns of mental health nurses. Good nursing leadership was seen as essential for the development of Mental Health Nursing against a background of change.

Recommendation 12
We recommend that immediate action is taken to improve the standard of management and leadership in Mental Health Nursing and mental health services.

Facilitating quality care

Quality assurance is a key issue for managers and practitioners alike. Nursing teams at all levels should have an explicit strategy for continuous improvements in standards of care. This requires that quality awareness and clinical audit should be integral to all service planning and included in pre-registration and continuing education programmes.

Mental Health Nursing Services should define specific standards for care and desired outcomes in partnership with people who use services. They should measure: the benefit of services to people; the responsiveness of the service to users; the extent to which the service addresses quality of life and caters for individual differences; and to what extent people who use services are involved in their planning.

The standard of care offered is dependent on the environment in which it is delivered. A therapeutic environment for high-quality Mental Health Nursing is one in which empathy, tolerance and support for others form an integral part of the workplace culture. Mental Health Nursing concerns itself with some of the most distressing aspects of human life and, as such, makes great demands on the individual. Therefore high-quality care is ultimately predicated on the compassionate management and adequate support of staff. Managers should respond imaginatively to retain mental health nurses at the relevant grades. For example, flexible working arrangements (part-time working, job-sharing and child care provision) are essential if more female nurses are to be promoted into senior clinical and managerial grades.

It is not enough to make advances in care. The Mental Health Nursing Service should be able to measure and demonstrate the added value which new thinking brings. It is also essential that managers recognise the efforts of their staff to improve quality of practice, and good practice should be celebrated and disseminated.

High priority should be given to the allocation of resources for research into the development of valid quality assurance systems and, at local level, we would like to see the systematic development of a range of quality assurance activities such as standard setting, clinical audit and user surveys.

Recommendation 13
We recommend that managers construct clear local strategies for Mental Health Nursing, developing a framework for good practice.

Multi-agency working

Comprehensive services demand comprehensive planning, and this depends on collaboration with other social and health care providers – including organisations responsible for housing provision. Clarity of relative responsibilities is essential and common protocols need to be established for referrals, assessment, care management and discharge. Joint agency working often raises issues of power and control over resources. However, whilst sovereignty clearly remains with the responsible authority, there should be shared accountability for the development of services based upon users' needs, rather than those of the agencies or the professionals.

Healthy boundaries should be established to protect professional integrity, but these should not be so rigid as to prevent work in differing settings. They should provide a framework to support the particular role, values and skills of mental health nurses.

Recommendation 14
We recommend that, in multi-disciplinary/agency working, managers should establish protocols which explicitly define the relative responsibilities of the various professionals involved.

Partnerships in care can be used to promote the formation of information systems to capture data which would identify needs, underpinning service planning and care planning review mechanisms. This would introduce more order into nursing practice and avoid reliance on ad hoc responses to crises or intuitive guesses about the nature of difficulties.

Consistent care for people with serious and enduring mental illness requires continuing effort and negotiation from both health and social services. Mental Health Nursing is valued in primary care settings both by general practitioners and community nurses, but it is important for providing agencies to specify the contracted function of mental health nurses in their employ. This specification should be set within established priorities, formal levels of activity and quality standards, so that nurses can focus on high-quality practice and adhere to contract specifications.

Recommendation 15
We recommend that commissioners and providers of mental health services should include Mental Health Nursing input when formulating, implementing and monitoring health care strategies.

2.3.4   **Liaison Mental Health Nursing**

We have found encouraging evidence of mental health nurses working in exciting and innovative ways in settings not always immediately associated with their specialty. Mental health nurses working in hospital accident and emergency departments with people who deliberately harm themselves were the pioneers of such work, which has now spread to include valuable liaison work in many areas of physical health. These nurses are delivering short-term interventions to people at times of distress, assessing the need for further referral and working to offer support to nursing colleagues, midwives and health visitors working in areas of high stress.

Mental health nurses have a valuable role to play in supporting other health and social care workers, especially in the development of assessment skills and care techniques for people with mental health problems who do not require specialist intervention.

Recommendation 16
We recommend the establishment of research programmes examining the potential of liaison Mental Health Nursing.

2.3.5   **Particular requirements of primary health care, a framework for collaboration**

Many mental health nurses are working within the context of primary health care and the continued development of general practitioner fundholders will be mirrored by an increase in the demand for the skills of mental health nurses. Individual general practitioners and the Royal College of General Practitioners emphasised the need for the expertise and the knowledge of mental health nurses in the primary care context.

A great deal of mental illness is treated in the community by general practitioners. Their understanding of the management of mental illness is uneven, but their demand to have mental health nurses working in the community grows constantly. The Review Team heard that a group of five general practitioners would have an average of 10,000 patients on their books. General practitioners suggested that this caseload warrants input from a mental health nurse on a full-time basis.

Increasingly, community care initiatives are resulting in the discharge of long-term residents with schizophrenia and other serious and enduring mental illnesses into the care of primary health teams. Referrals to mental health nurses working in the community from general practitioners have risen by 12.5% in the period 1985-90, so that they now almost equal the number of referrals from psychiatrists.[17]

It is important to continue a dialogue with general practitioners about care provision, especially given the number of exciting developments in primary care led by general practitioners, nurses and health visitors. The skills of the mental health nurse are an important resource for all members of the Primary Health Care team and should be directly accessible to the general public.

Mental health nurses will need to collaborate with colleagues in primary care to create protocols which address the mental health needs of the local community. It is, however, possible to provide a broader framework for the particular work of mental health nurses and their collaboration with midwives, health visitors, practice nurses and community nurses (*Figure 2*).

Figure 2

A suggested framework for collaborative working by Nurses, Midwives and Health Visitors in Mental Health Care

Location of Work

1 **Primary Prevention**
   Reducing the incidence of mental illness.
   (People at risk approximately 250 per thousand per year)

   Needs the work of Health Visitors, District Nurses, School Nurses, Practice Nurses and the specialist support of Mental Health Nurses.

   Work with vulnerable people or those at risk of mental illness

2 **Secondary Prevention**
   Early detection leading to prompt intervention.
   (People at risk approximately 100 per thousand per year)

   Needs the work of Health Visitors, District Nurses, School Nurses and Practice Nurses. Requires continuous liaison and some casework by Mental Health Nurses.

   Early detection and case finding, leading to early intervention. Work mostly carried out in the Primary Health Care Setting

3 **Tertiary Prevention**
   Treatment and active intervention with established mental illness. (People at risk approximately 24 per thousand per year).

   Needs the work of Mental Health Nurses in hospitals, residential facilities, day and community care. Needs liaison and work with Health Visitors, District Nurses, School Nurses and Practice Nurses.

   Early intervention effective treatment and rehabilitation requiring active case management

Recommendation 17

We recommend that Mental Health Nursing skills are available to all members of the Primary Health Care Team and are directly accessible to the general public.

There are of course other professionals on hand to offer skilled assistance. Psychologists and social workers have expressed a view that there is a need to identify client needs and to reach agreement on who has the skills to meet them. This underscores the importance of clarifying objectives and meshing the various professional contributions in an effective collaborative effort.

Such involvement will require that mental health nurses have a very clear understanding of the client group with whom they are primarily concerned, and the extent of their own input – direct and indirect – to primary health care provision.

Despite evidence of mature and predominantly good working relationships, there is evidence of some tension between what mental health nurses have attempted to provide and the expectations of other professional groups, particularly psychiatrists and general practitioners. This has led to confusion for people who use services and unsustainable demands on nurses by medical colleagues. We re-emphasise that mental health nurses should focus on people who have serious or enduring mental illness.

We look to the Care Programme Approach,[28] the new role of general practitioners as fund-holders, the key worker concept and a more active partnership with people who use services and their carers to counter these inter and intra-professional problems.

Evidence from people who use services emphasises the potential for the skills of nursing. As locally-based services for people with mental illness are developed further, the spotlight falls on the gap between primary and secondary care. Various individuals and groups felt that the people whose role most suitably bridges that gap are the mental health nurses working in the community: they would like to see nurses playing an important part in developing approaches which cross the divide between primary and secondary care.

2.3.6   **Care Programme Approach**

The Care Programme Approach, introduced in April 1991, involves collaboration between health and social services in order to provide individually-tailored care programmes for people with mental health problems newly accepted by specialist mental health services – and for people about to be discharged from a mental health hospital. Mental health nurses are increasingly being nominated as 'key workers', which means they are responsible for:

- *collaboration with service-users and their carers*

- *acting as a consistent point of contact for service-users, carers and other professionals*

- *ensuring that the user is registered with a GP and working in close contact with the primary health care team*

- *ensuring access to health promotion and chronic disease management at primary health care level*

- *being aware of other resources and referring appropriately*

- *planning and monitoring with others the delivery of the agreed care package, recording decisions made about it and ensuring regular review.*

There are still some problems with the understanding and implementation of the key worker principle in community mental health teams. We heard evidence of problems relating to clinical leadership and effective prioritisation of cases and resources. It is important that allocation of a key worker reflects the needs of the individual user of services and ensures that different professional skills are used to best effect. Effective team leadership is required to ensure equitable distribution of referrals and ongoing monitoring.

Supervised Discharge Planning

2.3.7

The Secretary of State for Health's recent package of measures[29] to reinforce good practice in the supervision and support for people when they leave hospital incorporates the principles of the Care Programme Approach, including a named key worker for each patient (*Figure 3*). The idea of developing a concept of 'supervised discharge' will meet with the support of the majority of mental health nurses; certainly there was sufficient evidence heard for it during the course of the review and some enthusiasm from nurses to act as key workers.

Figure 3

A ten point plan for successful and safe community care

1. **Strengthened powers to supervise the care of patients detained under the 1983 Mental Health Act who need special support after they leave hospital.**

   These comprise:

   - **the new power of supervised discharge; and**

   - **extending from six months to one year the period during which patients given extended leave under existing arrangements can be recalled to hospital.**

2. **Publication of the Department of Health team's report of its review of the 1983 Mental Health Act.**

3. **Publication of an improved version of the Code of Practice, which spells out clearly the criteria for compulsory admission under the 1983 Act.**

4. **Fresh guidance to ensure both that psychiatric patients are not discharged from hospital inappropriately, and that those who leave get the right support from the different agencies.**

5. **Better training for key workers in their duties under the care programme approach. This will cover the new Code of Practice and guidance, and will take account of the lessons from the cases which have gone wrong, and from the Royal College of Psychiatrists' confidential inquiry into homicides and suicides by mental ill people.**

6. **Encouraging the development of better information systems, including special supervision registers of patients who may be most at risk and need most support.**

7. **A review, by the Clinical Standards Advisory Group, of standards of care for people with schizophrenia, both in hospital and in the community.**

> 8 An agreed work programme for the Government's Mental Health Task Force, which supports health authorities in moving to locally-based care.
>
> 9 Ensuring the health authority and GP fund-holder purchasing plans cover the essential needs for mental health services.
>
> 10 The London Implementation Group will take forward an action programme to help improve mental health services in the capital, identifying and spreading best practice.

Recommendation 18

We recommend that action is taken to ensure that mental health nurses play a central role in services made available under the Care Programme Approach and in the provision of supervised discharge.

2.3.8

The changing demands of reprovision

There have been considerable advances in the reprovision of services which are acknowledged by this review. There are specific demands on nurses working in traditional psychiatric hospital settings: as the reprovision programme advances remaining hospital residents will become an increasingly focused and harder-to-place group, leaving the possibility that resources supporting them will diminish.

The Review Team have heard and seen evidence of creative and innovative work by mental health nurses both in preparing residents to leave institutional care and in trying to prepare themselves for evolving roles. Such creativity is by no means universal and there is a continuing demand for support and assistance for mental health nurses, as well as for residents who have to make this difficult transition. Mental health nurses have an individual professional responsibility to prepare themselves to work creatively with residents in advance of new service development, but this can only be done with sufficient personal and corporate support and education and training. (*See 2.6*)

Against a background of growing public and media concern about people with mental illness in the community, it is right that this review has examined the part nurses can play in ensuring that those who need treatment receive it appropriately and effectively. As the reprovision programme gathers pace in the last part of this century, greater emphasis will have to be placed on ensuring effective support systems for people with serious and enduring mental illness. We believe mental health nurses are well placed to provide such support in both the short and long term.

Recommendation 19

We recommend that the collective and individual needs of nurses presently working in large mental hospitals should be identified and met.

2.3.9

District general hospitals

Evidence presented to the Review Team suggests that changes are needed in the organisation of mental health services within district general hospitals. Many nurses considered the DGH unit had serious deficiencies as a therapeutic setting given the changes in patient mix. Nonetheless, nurses have risen to the challenge of working in these often unsuitable environments: we saw evidence of good work, despite deficiencies in design and location, where nurses had provided privacy, protection and therapeutic environments in centres not designed to provide them. We consider that design and location have a major part to play in the provision of care; working around deficiencies of design and location is an unnecessary distraction for mental health nurses.

It is thought that in-patient populations in district general hospital units are changing, with an increase in drug-related problems and aggressive or challenging behaviour. This challenges nursing staff who are required to balance the competing demands for care, making vulnerable residents feel safe while at the same time coping with difficult behaviour problems. The requirement for a 'standard' DGH Unit will change as providers and commissioners respond to the demands of local populations.

Recommendation 20
We recommend an urgent review of the therapeutic suitability of mental health units within district general hospitals.

2.4

Challenging issues facing mental health nurses

2.4.1

Gender and mental health

There is evidence to show that mental health services discriminate against women and do not adequately address their needs. Whilst more women than men are diagnosed as having mental health problems, men are much more likely to be referred for specialist help.[31] Women are also less likely than men to be identified by general practitioners as having mental health problems.

Mental health nurses are well placed to consider the overall needs and safety of women and to assist primary care colleagues in improving the recognition of mental health problems and the need for specialist help.

It is clear that sex role stereotypes of women are exerting an influence on the practice of Mental Health Nursing with consequences for both female service-users and female mental health nurses. We should ensure that assessment is sensitive to those issues which have been demonstrated to have a crucial bearing on the mental health of women, including: low self-esteem, reduced autonomy, male aggression and sexual abuse, emotional needs, social stress, poverty and low occupational status.

Only a comprehensive examination of women's needs as individuals can begin to ensure that services are effectively offering women choice and active involvement in their own care programme. As a priority, all mental health services should move to a situation in which the provision of single-sex accommodation and the choice of gender of named nurse or key worker is offered to all women. The Review Team noted with concern the findings of an analysis of data from the UKCC which indicate disproportionate numbers of disciplinary cases brought before the Council which involve male mental health nurses and female patients.

Recommendation 21
We recommend that mental health services develop a system offering a choice of single-sex accommodation and gender of a key worker.

2.4.2

Homeless and rootless people

Services should be taken to homeless and rootless people.[32] This may involve street work, working out of hours, and working with the criminal justice system – any of which may be unfamiliar territory for mental health nurses. People who are homeless are likely to have particular physical and social needs as well as mental health problems. Therefore, nurses should be able to collaborate effectively with primary care nurses and other agencies.

2.4.3

HIV and AIDS

The AIDS epidemic has challenged nurses' ability to accept the life-styles of others without stigma or prejudice. Associated as it is with sexual and drug-using behaviour, HIV disease

32

can expose affected individuals to discrimination and rejection.

The Review Team are aware of innovative educational initiatives in this field and of mental health nurses working very successfully with people with HIV/AIDS in some parts of the country. These nurses are also frequently involved in supporting staff in acute and palliative care settings who are dealing on a daily basis with the difficulties surrounding the disease and the deaths of those affected. Despite these educational initiatives and undoubted successes, there remains a continuing need for close monitoring of the response of mental health nurses to those suffering from HIV-related dementia.

It is essential that clinical managers closely monitor the response to the care of those with HIV-related mental health needs and deal sensitively and honestly with the fears and deficiencies of nursing staff. The mental health needs of partners, carers and family members also require particular attention. Recent work has suggested that a failure to recognise the grief reactions and depression present in young gay men who have suffered multiple bereavement is resulting in increased risk behaviour in this population.[33]

Mental health nurses are experienced in dealing with loss, depression, anxiety, confusion and dementia. These conditions are found in people with HIV disease and require the attention of skilled Mental Health Nursing.

Recommendation 22
We recommend a local review of the care currently being offered by mental health nurses to those suffering from HIV and other related diseases.

Sexuality and mental health

2.4.4

Mental health nurses should display an awareness that sexuality and its expression makes up a fundamental part of the human condition. Whilst some mental health problems such as depression can have the effect of reducing sexual activity, people with mental health problems do not suddenly become asexual upon diagnosis. It is important for mental health nurses to respond in an adult fashion to the needs for privacy and dignity in institutional settings, and to respect the right of service-users to choose those with whom they form close relationships. It is also essential that the mental health nurse protects vulnerable, confused and disinhibited people from humiliation, mockery and abuse.

Gay or bi-sexual men and women frequently find it difficult to express their needs openly, for fear of rejection and abuse. It is important that the dominant culture of mental health nursing is one in which people are accepted equally and sensitively, irrespective of their sexual orientation, and that the legitimacy of their partners is recognised.

Sexual abuse

2.4.5

The links between mental ill health and previous experience of sexual abuse are well known. Findings from a study by the London School of Economics (LSE) and Camberwell Health Authority would suggest that the issue of sexual abuse receives little attention in mental health services.[34] Studies have found that, although up to 40% of women in mental health services have been sexually abused as children, the majority of staff did not give a high priority to the issue of abuse;[35] [36] indeed, it is common for coping mechanisms to be misinterpreted as symptoms of pathology, and assessments are often made which ignore the context of abuse, thereby perpetuating the problem.

One problem in such cases is the failure of staff to believe that such events can occur. The benefit of the doubt will inevitably favour the abuser and it is all too common for such complaints to be written off as part of the 'illness'. The use of independent advocacy in these situations is of immense importance.

Relationships of great trust and intimacy can be, and sometimes are, exploited by staff working in the field of mental health. All mental health nurses require clear guidelines in order to be able to report incidents and deal with them sensitively but appropriately. The LSE/Camberwell study found no hospital with a policy or training programme covering sexual harassment or abuse. A code of practice for staff concerning the issue of sexual harassment and abuse is an essential priority.

Recommendation 23
We recommend that a code of practice covering the issue of sexual harassment and abuse is developed for staff providing mental health services.

2.4.6

Care of elderly people

The proportion of older people in our society is increasing all the time: in the United Kingdom, the percentage of those over 65 has trebled since the beginning of the century. By the year 2001, there will be an increase of 4% in those over 65, of 20% among those aged 75-79, and of 31% in those aged 80-84, with a 46% increase in those older still. The chance of admission to a psychiatric hospital is greatly increased in later life with approximately one in four adults admitted being over 65. Research indicates that this is only the tip of the iceberg, as the vast majority of mental health problems among elderly people are managed by carers in the home. Whilst many older people are cared for with great dedication by the primary health care team and their families, there are many others who fail to draw attention to their need for services.

The *Mental Illness Key Area Handbook* notes that suicide among the elderly population remains very high.[37] Depressive illness is the most treatable and the most common mental health problem in those over 65, with up to 10% suffering significant depression which interferes with functioning. Evidence would suggest that such depression is frequently not recognised and, even when correctly diagnosed, is treated in a limited manner resulting in high relapse and poor recovery rates. Mental health nurses have a crucial role to play in improving the care for elderly people who are often suffering unnecessarily.[38]

Mental health nurses working with elderly people perform invaluable work, but we found evidence of under-investment in training, support and supervision for nursing staff in relation to the very complex and demanding needs of those suffering from dementia. It is especially important for mental health nurses to be aware that elderly people and their carers have access to a comprehensive range of services which take into account their physical and mental health needs.

Co-ordination of care is a particular concern, because care is invariably provided by a multiplicity of agencies, both statutory and non-statutory. Care outside the hospital or residential setting relies heavily upon the goodwill and hard work of carers, and they should be fully involved in a dialogue with providers and commissioners if elderly people suffering from dementia are to have a voice. The challenge for mental health nurses is to deliver the highest level of care whilst at the same time vigorously protecting the right of the elderly person with dementia to maintain as much independence as possible for as long as possible.

Recommendation 24

We recommend a local review of arrangements of the support and supervision of nurses working with elderly people with mental illness by Commissioners and Providers of services.

Mental health of children and adolescents

2.4.7

Mental health problems in children and adolescents are likely to persist in later life if left untreated. Evidence suggests that assessments are often complex and many GPs are failing to detect such children and young people.[31] Thorough investigation is often required – of the family situation as well as the child's own problems. It is also necessary to assess the young person's physical health and development. The Review Team wish to acknowledge the valuable work being undertaken by health visitors, school nurses and other professional colleagues. Such involvement with emotionally disturbed children and young people calls for a high degree of multi-disciplinary teamwork, with mental health nurses playing a vital role.

During the course of the review, we heard of services in crisis as professionals and agencies involved in providing district-based services reorganise and redeploy their resources. We were informed, for example, that social workers have been re-allocated to child protection teams to fulfil local authority responsibilities under *The Children Act* (1989). This has led to increased demand on school nurses, health visitors and mental health nurses.

The Review Team are aware of the review of the commissioning and management of mental health services for children and adolescents currently being undertaken by the Health Advisory Service. Such an examination of the service is timely and important in providing commissioning agencies with appropriate guidance.

Recommendation 25

We recommend a local review of the role and function of mental health nurses working in child and adolescent mental health services, with a view to enabling them to work more effectively alongside their nursing colleagues, other disciplines and agencies.

Substance misuse

2.4.8

Substance misuse is not an illness, but rather a range of behaviours that have a major impact on the wellbeing of the individual and society. It is directly implicated in a high proportion of suicides, unplanned pregnancies, cancers, heart conditions, HIV transmission and poor mental health. In their role of promoting behavioural changes, mental health nurses have a major contribution to make in achieving the targets set in the report, *Health of the Nation*.[9] They have a key role to play in primary prevention, initiating early intervention strategies and engaging clients in harm reduction measures, treatment and rehabilitation, and relapse prevention.

Mental health nurses with specialist skills in this area are an essential resource to other care workers who encounter people with substance misuse problems daily in the performance of their duties. Whilst there is no doubt that many acute or long-term problems will continue to need the input of specialists, all mental health nurses should be capable of prevention, recognition and early intervention. Such skills are important in many areas of Mental Health Nursing and there is an urgent need to disseminate the many excellent examples of innovative work in this field to all nurses in mental health and others in the primary health care teams. It is also increasingly important for mental health nurses to make links with all sections of the criminal justice system.

2.4.9

Mentally disordered offenders

Services for mentally disordered offenders have been made a first-order priority for the NHS 1994/95 (EL(93)54). This requires NHS authorities to work with personal social services and criminal justice agencies to develop strategic and purchasing plans for services for mentally disordered offenders.

It follows the review of health and social services for mentally disordered offenders[39] [40] and the view expressed in *Care Custody and Justice* that: "*Prison is not a suitable place for people suffering from serious mental disturbance*".[41] These reports emphasise the importance of prompt identification and assessment of offenders suspected of suffering from mental disorder, and diversion from the criminal justice system.

In the past, mental health nurses working in secure environments have been isolated from their colleagues working in other settings. There is now a need for greater interaction and sharing of knowledge and skills in practice, research and education.

Nurses working with mentally disordered offenders have to deal with their own feelings, fears and judgements and cope with morbid public curiosity and media attention. Most importantly, they should manage the apparent contradictions involved in empowering such individuals by working with high levels of therapeutic skill in a secure environment.

Recommendation 26
We recommend that greater links are forged between mental health nurses working in substance misuse and services for mentally disordered offenders, and the criminal justice system.

2.4.10

Risk assessment

There is no doubt that, for the majority of users of mental health services (particularly those people who were formerly residents of large mental hospitals), the move to community care and increased normalisation has brought great benefits. Even though the merits of community care are now clearly demonstrated, there are real concerns about the risk which a small proportion of people with serious mental health problems might pose in the community. This has been focused on a small, but tragic number of high-profile incidents of violence and suicide, prompting an internal review by Secretary of State for Health of the care of vulnerable people with mental health problems who might slip through the net of services.

To date, much of the 'risk assessment' undertaken by mental health nurses has been intuitive and informal. The implementation of the care programme approach – involving a named key worker – will require mental health nurses to offer more formal specifications of their risk assessment methods, including the criteria underpinning clinical judgements. Many of the groups mentioned in the preceding sections are known to be more vulnerable to mental illness. There is an urgent need to review current practice and to define methods which identify individuals 'at risk', as well as delivering programmes to deliver effective, appropriate intervention and support strategies.

Mental health nurses and research

The complex nature of mental health and mental illness means that research is not a simple task. For the purposes of this review, research is defined as follows:

"We use the term research to mean rigorous and systematic enquiry, conducted on a scale and using methods commensurate with the issue to be investigated, and designed to lead to more generalised contributions to knowledge."

Within this general definition, the focus of this review is on research by nurses and others into Mental Health Nursing, the wider field of general psychiatry and the general arena of service delivery. The Review Team recognise that not all mental health nurses will wish to be (or are equipped to be) active in research. However, we believe that all nurses should be research-literate. We should also recognise the contribution that mental health nurses can make to research activity in general.

There is some encouraging evidence that nurses can conduct high-quality research in all these areas. Graduate and postgraduate programmes are providing useful research material. Mental health nurses are also competing with some success for research funds. However, there is no room for complacency. Having demonstrated the capacity to produce good work, Mental Health Nursing needs encouragement, resources and strategic planning to achieve its potential as a generator of valuable research.

Recommendation 27
We recommend that managers invest in the continuing development of the research skills base among mental health nurses through a series of positive steps related to funded support.

Research: the policy push

There has been considerable policy activity which has stimulated research attempting to answer questions about the delivery of health care and the relative contributions of single- and multi-disciplinary effort. Department of Health and Regional Research and Development Committees have research agendas which include priorities related to mental illness.[42] Mental health nurses have a substantial part to play in this by contributing to research into mental health services generally, Mental Health Nursing specifically, and the effectiveness of care delivered to people who use services. The *Key Area Handbook for Mental Illness* clearly identifies research responsibilities for service-providers. More recently, *A Strategy for Research in Nursing*[43] has provided a greater sense of focus and direction for research activity by nurses, midwives and health visitors.

Recommendation 28
We recommend that Regional Research and Development Committees define the action they are taking to respond to the recommendations of the Task Force on the Strategy for Research in Nursing Midwifery and Health Visiting, with particular reference to Mental Health Nursing.

2.5.2 **Providing an academic base for mental health nurse researchers**

Graduate mental health nurses are already emerging from a number of university courses and further programmes are planned. Two centres provide accelerated registration programmes for graduates. A supply of potential researchers can be drawn from these programmes and a number already go on to receive postgraduate studentships or to work as university researchers.

Many other mental health nurses are obtaining graduate and postgraduate awards on a full- or part-time basis, from a variety of subject programmes. It is important to note that some badly supervised, student-led studies are of a poor quality and, as such, are damaging the potential for more properly constructed research. It is hoped that those learning research can be encouraged to do so in *'laboratory conditions'* and not in the field, where mistakes can be damaging. The location of nurse education in universities, the attendant benefits of the research culture and schemes such as credit accumulation and transfer, have all been to the advantage of Mental Health Nursing.

2.5.3 **Developing centres of research activity**

A number of mental health nurses have received financial support to undertake research. However, it has been reported repeatedly to this review that there are problems finding an academic centre either conducting research related to Mental Health Nursing or willing to support a prospective researcher. We do not have an accurate figure for the number of centres with either declared or actual expertise in research into Mental Health Nursing. However, the last Higher Education Funding Council research exercise indicates that they are few in number and do not receive substantial funding.

A number of professors of nursing in the UK are reported to have a declared interest and visible expertise in Mental Health Nursing research. It is encouraging that prospective researchers now have a growing choice of sites where they can conduct their own research under sympathetic and knowledgeable supervision. Hopefully, the expertise of such centres will continue to become more publicly known through completed work and published papers. Clearly, university-based departments of nursing are not the only points at which research into Mental Health Nursing will take place. Nevertheless, there is a need to establish a *'critical mass'*[44] of research activity by nurses if a research culture is to be established in Mental Health Nursing.

Research activities closely related to Mental Health Nursing have received some funding support from central sources, and although there is now no separately identified budget for nursing research, the Department of Health has commissioned research which does involve mental health nurses.

A survey among academic departments to investigate declared interest in research methods, skills and opportunities would provide a clearer picture of the current situation and the need for investment.

Recommendation 29
We recommend that the Central Research and Development Division of the Department of Health identifies what Mental Health Nursing research resources are at its disposal.

Research by mental health nurses 2.5.4

The report *Psychiatric Nursing: Today and Tomorrow* (1968) on Mental Health Nursing predicted a rise in research by British mental health nurses – as had been seen in America. A number of priorities for research were identified, many of which have been explored but all of which warrant further study today. These research areas include: working in hospitals as against the community; studies of good administrative practice; studies of Mental Health Nursing practice; research into the psychotherapeutic role of the nurse; relieving nurses of non-nursing duties; identifying standards of care and associated staffing levels. *Better Services for the Mentally Ill* (1975) identified as priorities for research: new long-stay patients; care of elderly mentally ill people; support and advice for relatives; skill mix studies; and evaluations of different treatment approaches.[45]

The development of a body of research into Mental Health Nursing has been slow but is showing some recent signs of growth. There have been comments on the paucity of research on Mental Health Nursing,[46] and some which stress the need for a body of knowledge on which to base practice.[47] There have been advances in research design, in subject focus[48] and in multi-disciplinary approaches.[3] [4]

Mental health nurses and multi-disciplinary research 2.5.5

There is growing emphasis on the importance of multi-disciplinary research, and there are centres to be funded which will be based around multi-disciplinary research teams. Mental health nurses should play their part in this, but their relative inexperience compared to other disciplines may be a disadvantage.

However, examples of competent and sometimes nurse-led collaborative activities were provided to the Review Team. The Thorn Nurse initiative in London and Manchester, designed to prepare and evaluate the work of mental health nurses with people who have schizophrenia, is the product of a number of research strands from nursing, psychology and psychiatry. It has produced a research-based programme to help mental health nurses work specifically with people who have schizophrenia. Work by nurses and health economists has been reported, and also studies of primary care and community psychiatric nursing.[49]

Concerns were expressed about the diminishing resources in the clinical setting – particularly a lack of journals or research advice. It was clear that, as colleges of nursing have drawn together in large collegiate groups, they have become more distant from the clinical environment, making access to libraries and academic help more difficult.

Research needs the right conditions to flourish: positioning libraries and databases in locations remote from clinical areas is unlikely to encourage people to inform their practice with the latest research findings. Creative solutions to such problems were cited including remote computer terminals within clinical areas which were connected to libraries and databases. MIDIRS (Midwives' Information Resource Service) is a subscription circulation which gives the latest information on research and development in midwifery, and it was suggested that a similar system should be created for Mental Health Nursing.

Recommendation 30
We recommend that a version of the Midwives' Information Resource Service (MIDIRS) should be established for Mental Health Nursing.

2.6

Mental health nursing: initial and continuing education

2.6.1

Pre-registration education programmes

The title 'registered nurse' is protected by law and a Register of Nurses is maintained by the United Kingdom Central Council for Nursing, Midwifery and Health Visiting (UKCC).[50] Entry to the Register is permitted only on successful completion of a programme approved by the appropriate National Board for Nursing, Midwifery and Health Visiting in the United Kingdom. Under the current scheme – Project 2000 – pre-registration education and training for all nurses now leads to a Diploma in Higher Education and registration on the appropriate part of the Professional Register maintained by the UKCC.

The first half of the three-year pre-registration programme comprises a Common Foundation Programme (CFP) which is undertaken by all students, irrespective of their subsequent specialisation. This is followed by an eighteen-month Branch Programme of specialisation in either Adult, Mental Health, Learning Disability or Children's Nursing. In Mental Health Nursing this has superseded a three-year programme leading to the Registered Mental Nurse (RMN) qualification.

All pre-registration and virtually all post-registration education and training is provided by Colleges of Nursing/Midwifery/Health Studies and Institutes of Higher Education. Increasingly, Colleges of Nursing/Midwifery/Health Studies are integrating with the higher education sector.

Students receive credits for study through the increasing application of credit accumulation and transfer schemes to professional education and training. Recognition of relevant previous learning is taken into account, thus avoiding wasteful repetition of study.

Education and training provision is commissioned by service providers under arrangements set out in the Department of Health's paper: *Working for Patients: Education and Training Working Paper 10* (1989).[51] This arrangement ensures that education and training providers develop only those courses and modules for which there is a market, and in modes suitable to practitioners. Such arrangements have yet to have their full impact on the provision of education and training for nurses, midwives and health visitors.

2.6.2

Major issues facing pre-registration education

Pre-registration education and training aim to prepare competent practitioners who possess a set of core skills which enable them to care for people with either acute or long-term mental health problems; to assess, plan, implement and evaluate such care; to move confidently between hospital and community settings; and to acquire the necessary skills and knowledge to act as a key worker.

Project 2000 aims to provide a broader and deeper knowledge base than previous courses. The programme promises to deliver a knowledgeable, questioning and highly adaptable practitioner, able to analyse situations and respond appropriately. The versatility of the Project 2000 nurse should be especially valuable to services which are evolving rapidly to meet changing needs in society.

Three major issues were identified by the many contributors to the review as being relevant to the development and delivery of pre-registration programmes in Mental Health Nursing. These are:

- the perceived limitations of current education and training programmes

- the move from hospital to non-institutional settings

- the needs of people suffering from serious or enduring mental health problems.

Concerns about Project 2000   2.6.3

In evidence to the review, there was widespread concern that the new programme is not enabling students to develop sufficiently the essential skills of Mental Health Nursing. Many people feel that the balance of subjects within the CFP is wrong and gives insufficient emphasis to the core skills of the mental health nurse early in the programme.

It is important that the new programme maintains the discipline of Mental Health Nursing as a central focus. There were many calls for the length of the Branch Programme to be increased at the expense of the Common Foundation Programme. There was also a criticism that, in many instances, the clinical placements were not long enough to be educationally valuable.

Recommendation 31
We recommend that the Statutory Bodies review the balance of time and emphasis given to each of the four branch programmes within the Common Foundation Programme.

Students in the majority of course centres have to choose their branch programme at the beginning of the course. The original intention had been to allow students a choice at the end of the CFP, an approach supported by this review.

Against these vocal criticisms, others support the new programme, at least in terms of its intentions. Any comparison between the previous three-year mental nursing programme and the new programme should be made with caution. The two courses were not designed to achieve the same outcomes and so comparisons are not meaningful. The fact that it is too soon to identify the benefits of the new programme does not mean they do not exist; we should also remember the problems inherent in the previous system which led to the creation of Project 2000.

Education in practice   2.6.4

Students need to be exposed to a climate in which mental health nursing is valued. This climate of professional esteem should be positively fostered by educators and practitioners and form a key focus for students' own evaluations of their educational experience. The results of such evaluations should be widely distributed, discussed and acted upon. However, evidence indicates that educators are not making their mark within the Common Foundation Programme and, as a result, students are not always exposed to a culture in which Mental Health Nursing is valued.

Project 2000 seeks to prepare people to work in all settings. Nonetheless, there is evidence that newly qualified nurses are encouraged to work within an institution before moving into the community. Such practice will not test whether the new programme adequately prepares students to work safely in community settings.

A constant theme in the evidence to the review was the need to involve people who use services and their carers in all aspects of care and treatment, including the provision of education and training. Although no consensus exists on how this should be achieved, it is considered that it should be determined at local level. Those involved in providing courses need to demonstrate a commitment to enabling people who use services and their carers to make a meaningful contribution to education and training by including them as trainers in all courses. Such courses should be based on an assessment of user need, and might be based around the advanced skills of care management, including risk assessment. It is recognised that it may take some time for them to develop this aspect of their role and they will need support in the process.

Recommendation 32
We recommend that people who use services and their carers should participate in teaching and curriculum development.

There is an important corollary to the previous recommendation. Carers, and those groups representing carers, gain a great deal of support from mental health nurses. Consideration should be given to extending appropriate elements of education and training to carers, helping them to acquire appropriate knowledge and skills.

Nurse teachers can become isolated from the practice they teach. In a practice-led profession, which is facing such immense challenges, it is vital that education and training be delivered by people whose skills and knowledge are current and informed by an understanding of the pressures on practitioners. One interesting development is the appointment of teachers to the post of Lecturer/Practitioner.

There was much support from all quarters for nurse teachers to maintain their skills and knowledge in the practice of Mental Health Nursing, by spending the equivalent of one day a week in practice. How this is achieved should be determined locally and could include a range of possibilities. Equally, there is a need for practitioners to contribute more fully to the education and training function. Teaching staff and clinical practitioners require adequate professional development for their evolving educational roles.

Recommendation 33
We recommend that teachers of Mental Health Nursing should spend the equivalent of at least one day per week in practice to maintain the currency of their skills and knowledge.

2.6.5
Educational focus on special needs

All mental health nurses require an awareness of those groups of people within society who are particularly vulnerable in terms of their mental health. These include people who are homeless, unemployed, elderly and people with learning disabilities. In addition, education and training programmes need to address the specific issues within the profile of the local community. Courses should develop the student's ability to work with elderly people, children and people who exhibit challenging behaviour. Newly qualified mental health nurses should also possess basic skills in counselling and care management, and the ability to work as key members of the multi-disciplinary team.

Recommendation 34
We recommend that pre-registration education and training programmes ensure that students develop an awareness of the needs of those groups of people who are particularly vulnerable, such as homeless, unemployed and elderly people.

Programmes at both pre- and post-registration levels should include a focus on the special needs of black and ethnic minority groups.

Recommendation 35
We recommend that all education and training programmes reflect the diversity of belief systems and cultural expectations that contribute to the life experience of people who use services.

Concerns about recruitment   2.6.6

Figures published by the English National Board (*Annex E*), indicate an alarming reduction of over 50% in the number of initial entries and re-entries to Mental Health Nursing education and training in the six years 1981/82 (3995) to 1987/88 (1990). Over the last five years to 1992/93 the numbers have levelled out, but they are now beginning to fall again.

When the numbers of post-registration student entries (that is practitioners already registered on another part of the Professional Register) are added to the equation, the picture is less dramatic, with a fall of 12.4% over the eight years 1984/85 (3457) to 1992/93 (3028). A major reason for this is the large number of second-level nurses who have become first-level mental health practitioners in recent years. It should be remembered however, that such 'conversion' has not contributed to the overall pool of mental health nurses.

It is difficult to anticipate accurately the kind of workforce needed in future. The length of the preparation period indicates a need to recruit the right number of students today to provide enough qualified nurses in three to four years' time. Evidence that commissioners are opting for short-term contracts for service provision (one-year rolling programmes, for example) makes long-term planning even more problematic.

Some factors (such as changes in the mix of mental health workers) clearly indicate a need to reduce training numbers. However, these are countered by factors which, though less obvious, argue strongly for an increase in numbers. These include the growing demand for mental health nurses within the developing private and voluntary sectors, the implications of the report on the *Review of Health and Social Services for Mentally Disordered Offenders and Others Requiring Similar Services*, and the high morbidity of mental health problems within the general population. Recent decisions by provider units to commission fewer student places on pre-registration Mental Health Nursing programmes show a lack of foresight and could well result in a shortfall in the near future.

Recommendation 36
We recommend a systematic national review of strategic planning to ensure that training commissions accurately reflect service needs.

The contribution to service   2.6.7

It was originally hoped that students undertaking the new Project 2000 programmes would enjoy full student status throughout. However, the replacement costs for the loss of the service contribution previously provided by students in traditional apprentice-type training were substantial. In the final proposals for Project 2000, the UKCC acknowledged the high practical content of the programme, with students making a significant contribution to service.[52] The Central Council went on to say that this service contribution could be recognised as part of the programme, as long as it was educationally determined. It was eventually considered that a service contribution of 20% of the total programme (ie 1000 hours), was appropriate and that this should preferably be undertaken in the third year. This has led to difficulties.

The funding arrangements necessary to account for this service contribution differ across the country. However, organising the payment can significantly restrict the opportunities for educationally-led clinical experience. This is of particular concern within the Mental Health Branch because many pre-Project 2000 mental health courses had previously achieved a position where little or none of the clinical experience contributed to service for accounting purposes.

In addition, there is anecdotal evidence that a reliance on the rostered contribution of Adult Nursing students has had a detrimental effect on recruitment to other branches of nursing in some centres. In other words, there is a greater commitment to recruiting students to the Adult Nursing Branch because they continue to provide so much care during their rostered periods of service.

Recommendation 37
We recommend that the period of rostered service within Project 2000 nursing programmes be discontinued.

2.6.8   **Continuing professional development and specialist education**

Qualified mental health nurses are required to keep up to date through continuing professional development. Yet the availability of specific courses for mental health nurses at post-registration level is limited, and has improved little since this deficit was highlighted by the former Joint Board of Clinical Nursing Studies (JBCNS) in 1978. In England, the newly developed Framework and Higher Award now provides an opportunity for commissioners of education and training to ensure that practitioners develop the required skills through the provision of appropriate courses and modules.[53] This should also increase the opportunities for continuing professional development through the establishment of pathways leading to the Higher Award of the English National Board.

Recommendation 38
We recommend that particular and appropriate education and training at post-registration level is made available to all mental health nurses.

The delivery of post-registration mental health nursing courses and modules should integrate college-based study with practice. This can be facilitated by more flexible and cost-effective learning packages utilising open, distance and self-directed learning.

With the convergence of professional education into institutes of higher education, the opportunities for shared learning and joint educational initiatives between health care professionals should increase. Appropriate shared learning will also enable more cost-effective use of resources and facilities. The development of multi-agency working in practice should also provide a stimulus for such initiatives.

Given the extent of mental health problems in the community and the limited number of mental health nurses, there is a clear need for the mental health training component of non-mental health nurses to be reviewed and strengthened. In addition, mental health nurses need to develop their role in relation to other care workers. For example, mental health nurses could play a greater role in helping colleagues to develop the assessment skills required to identify when onward referral is necessary. They could also help other health care workers to provide appropriate support for people who do not need the expertise of a specialist practitioner.

Recommendation 39

We recommend that education providers should collaborate with service providers to develop further cost-effective shared learning packages which meet the needs of mental health nurses, other professionals and non-professional health care workers.

The need to invest in post-registration education and training to develop mental health nurses as specialists is acknowledged. As well as developing specific clinical skills, it will be increasingly necessary to develop expertise related to the changing context of health care delivery. Such skills include, for example, contract negotiation, risk assessment, and care management techniques.

Training budgets are notoriously vulnerable to cuts or redirection when funding is insufficient. The arrangements for purchasing education and training under *Working for Patients: Education and Training Paper 10* provides the opportunity to influence the range and quality of education provided, as well as the grade and skill-mix of nursing staff. This provision should be safeguarded for the purpose for which it was intended, that is education and training.

Recommendation 40

We recommend that action is taken to safeguard money available under Working Paper 10 arrangements.

The review found widespread support for provision of clinical supervision for all mental health nurses. (*See also Section 2.2*). Unlike a number of other professions, clinical supervision is not part of the culture of nursing. Therefore, not only do we need to prepare people to undertake a supervisory role, we also need to ensure nurses know what to expect from such supervision.

Recommendation 41

We recommend that new training initiatives aimed at developing clinical supervision skills in senior clinical nurses are devised. We also recommend that newly qualified nurses and nursing students receive preparation in what to expect from clinical supervision.

Although there is increasing emphasis on nursing skills in the community, there are various skill developments appropriate for nurses who will remain in hospital settings. These include counselling skills, management of the environment and related financial aspects, as well as the skills required for the Care Programme Approach described earlier.

Practitioners who care for people in large mental hospitals require re-training in order to develop skills more appropriate to care provided in community settings. Evidence was received that the re-training element of reprovision is not always given due attention. Employers and providers should be prepared to invest in the development of their qualified staff, and decisions about funding should not be based on short-term imperatives. (*See Section 2.3*). This is an important element of continuing professional development.

2.6.9

National Vocational Qualifications

The Care Sector Consortium, established in 1988, was one of the first Industry Lead Bodies. It has been responsible for the development of National Vocational Qualifications within the health and social care sector at Levels I to III.[54]

The more recently established Occupational Standards Council (OSC) for Health and Social Care has initiated a project to produce a full functional map of the care sector at all levels.[55] The OSC works with regulatory and statutory bodies to articulate the employment requirements for a competent workforce and thereby improve the quality of care to individuals. It is expected that NVQs at Levels IV & V will be developed.

In 1992, the UKCC approved the Level III National Vocational Qualification (NVQ) in health care as an entry gate to nurse education programmes leading to registration.[56] Shared understanding, a distillation of best practice and the co-ordination of occupational standards have already proved beneficial across the whole health care sector. Further work is needed to explore issues surrounding higher level vocational qualifications, but this should not deter the further identification of occupational standards.

Evidence to the Review Team suggested that the general principle of accreditation of prior learning, already applied to education and training at post-registration level, should be introduced within pre-registration education and training provision.

Recommendation 42
We recommend that the United Kingdom Central Council for Nursing, Midwifery and Health Visiting considers the accreditation of appropriate prior learning for entrants to pre-registration programmes.

"Mental health nursing should re-examine

3.0 THE WAY FORWARD

every aspect of its policy and practice

in the light of the needs of people

who use services."

3.1

Recommendations for progress

"The principle of choice for people who use services and their carers needs to be fully established as a basis for the practice of mental health nursing."

We noted at the beginning of this report that the work of mental health nurses rests upon the relationship they have with people who use services. Our recommendations for future action start and finish with this relationship.

If we had to sum up our report in one recommendation, it would be that, *"Mental health nursing should re-examine every aspect of its policy and practice in the light of the needs of people who use services"*. Nursing services should be designed and developed to meet the needs of people who use services: people should not be expected to conform to the convenience of the service.

Mental Health Nursing faces immense challenges in helping to meet the mental health needs of society. But we also believe that this is a period of great opportunity. Nurses need to foster a more constructive relationship with people who use services; they need to capitalise on the potential of multi-agency approaches to care; and they need to acquire advanced and specialised skills to play a full part in the multi-disciplinary team.

In rising to these challenges, mental health nurses will consolidate their position as key contributors to progressive mental health services. This will bring greater professional rewards to the individual practitioner and, more importantly, it will bring major advances in the quality of care. Our vision for the future of mental health services places mental health nurses in the vanguard of practice: building on existing expertise and developing new skills; collaborating confidently and constructively with colleagues in the multi-disciplinary team; and responding directly and appropriately to the needs of people who use services.

Implementing recommendations

R1   *We recommend that nurses improve their understanding and awareness of the racial and cultural needs of people who use services and ensure that these are fully reflected when developing care plans.*

Lead action by   Commissioners and Providers of Education & Training/ Mental Health Nurses

R2   *We recommend that mental health nurses take a lead role in ensuring that people in their care have access to appropriate information, including treatment options and rights.*

Lead action by   Mental Health Nurses/Providers of mental health services

R3   *We recommend that managers introduce a system of holding and acting upon information about people's wishes and needs in crisis.*

Lead action by   Providers of mental health services

R4   *We recommend the representation and participation of people who use services and their carers on service planning, education and research groups.*

Lead action by   Commissioners and Providers of mental health services

R5   *We recommend that the UKCC investigates and reports on the disproportionate numbers of disciplinary cases which involve male nurses and female patients*

Lead action by   UKCC

R6   *We recommend that the essential focus for the work of mental health nurses lies in working with people with serious or enduring mental illness in secondary and tertiary care, regardless of setting.*

Lead action by   Commissioners, GPs and Providers of mental health services

R7   *We recommend that Mental Health Nursing should retain its specialty at initial preparation level.*

Lead action by   UKCC

R8   *We recommend that care plans should be developed with individuals and based on their wishes and needs – not the convenience of the service.*

Lead action by   Commissioners and Providers of mental health services/ Mental Health Nurses

R9   *We recommend that Mental Health Nursing services should be arranged to ensure that nurses spend the majority of their time responding to the needs of people who use services.*

Lead action by   Providers of mental health services/Mental Health Nurses

R10   *We recommend that the title 'mental health nurse' be used both for nurses who work in the community and for those who work in hospital and day services.*

Lead action by   All

R11   *We recommend that clinical supervision is established as an integral part of practice up to and including the level of advanced practitioner for mental health nurses.*

Lead action by   Commissioners and Providers of mental health services

R12   *We recommend that immediate action is taken to improve the standard of management and leadership in Mental Health Nursing and mental health services.*

Lead action by   Department of Health/Commissioners and Providers of mental health services

R13   *We recommend that managers construct clear local strategies for Mental Health Nursing, developing a framework for good practice.*

Lead action by   Providers of mental health services

R14   *We recommend that, in multi-disciplinary/agency working, managers should establish protocols which explicitly define the relative responsibilities of the various professionals involved.*

Lead action by   Providers of mental health services/Mental Health Nurses

R15   *We recommend that commissioners and providers of mental health services include Mental Health Nursing input when formulating, implementing and monitoring health care strategies.*

Lead action by   Commissioners of mental health services

R16   *We recommend the establishment of research programmes to examine the potential of liaison mental health nursing.*

Lead action by   Department of Health/NHSME/RHAs

R17   *We recommend that Mental Health Nursing skills are available to all members of the Primary Health Care Team and are directly accessible to the general public.*

Lead action by   Commissioners and Providers of mental health services/Mental Health Nurses

R18   *We recommend that action is taken to ensure that mental health nurses play a central role in services made available under the Care Programme Approach and in the provision of supervised discharge.*

Lead action by   Commissioners and Providers of mental health services/
Mental Health Nurses

R19   *We recommend that the collective and individual needs of nurses presently working in large mental hospitals should be identified and met.*

Lead action by   Providers of mental health services/Commissioners of Education
& Training

R20   *We recommend an urgent review of the therapeutic suitability of district general hospital mental health units.*

Lead action by   Commissioners and Providers of mental health services

R21   *We recommend that mental health services develop a system offering a choice of single-sex accommodation and gender of a key worker.*

Lead action by   Commissioners and Providers of mental health services/Mental Health
Nurses

R22   *We recommend a local review of the care currently being offered by mental health nurses to those suffering from HIV and other related diseases.*

Lead action by   Commissioners and Providers of mental health services

R23   *We recommend that a code of practice covering the issue of sexual harassment and abuse is developed for staff providing mental health services.*

Lead action by   Commissioners and Providers of mental health services

R24   *We recommend a local review of arrangements of the support and supervision of nurses working with elderly people with mental illness by commissioners and providers of mental health services.*

Lead action by   Commissioners and Providers of mental health services

R25   *We recommend a local review of the role and function of mental health nurses working in child and adolescent mental health services, with a view to enabling them to work effectively alongside their colleagues, other disciplines and agencies.*

Lead action by   Commissioners and Providers of mental health services

R26   *We recommend that greater links are forged between mental health nurses working in substance misuse and services for mentally disordered offenders, and the criminal justice system.*

Lead action by   Department of Health/Home Office/Commissioners and Providers
of Mental Health Services/Mental Health Nurses

R27   *We recommend that managers invest in the continuing development of the research skills base among mental health nurses through a series of positive steps related to funded support.*

Lead action by   Providers of mental health services

R28   *We recommend that Regional Research and Development Committees define the action they are taking to respond to the recommendations of the Task Force on the Strategy for Research in Nursing, Midwifery and Health Visiting, with particular reference to Mental Health Nursing.*

Lead action by   Regional Research & Development Committees

R29   *We recommend that the Research and Development Division of the Department of Health identifies what Mental Health Nursing research resources are at its disposal.*

Lead action by   Department of Health Research and Development Directorate

R30   *We recommend that a version of the Midwives Information Resource Service (MIDIRS) should be established for Mental Health Nursing.*

Lead action by   Department of Health

R31   *We recommend that the Statutory Bodies review the balance of time and emphasis given to each of the four branches within the Common Foundation Programme.*

Lead action by   UKCC/ENB

R32   *We recommend that people who use services and their carers should participate in teaching and curriculum development.*

Lead action by   ENB/Commissioners and Providers of Education & Training

R33   *We recommend that teachers of Mental Health Nursing should spend the equivalent of at least one day per week in practice to maintain the currency of their skills and knowledge.*

Lead action by   Providers of Education & Training Faculty Heads

R34   *We recommend that pre-registration education and training programmes ensure that students develop an awareness of the needs of those groups of people who are particularly vulnerable, such as homeless, unemployed and elderly people.*

Lead action by   Providers of Education & Training/ENB

R35   *We recommend that all education and training programmes reflect the diversity of belief systems and cultural expectations that contribute to the life experience of people who use services.*

Lead action by   ENB/Commissioners of Education & Training/Providers of mental health services

R36   *We recommend a systematic national review of strategic planning to ensure that training commissions accurately reflect service needs.*

Lead action by   NHSME

R37   *We recommend that the period of rostered service within Project 2000 nursing programmes be discontinued.*

Lead action by   NHSME

R38   *We recommend that particular and appropriate education and training at post-registration level is made available for all mental health nurses.*

Lead action by   Commissioners and Providers of Education & Training

R39   *We recommend that education providers should collaborate with service providers to develop further cost-effective shared learning packages which meet the needs of mental health nurses, other professionals and non-professional health care workers.*

Lead action by   RHAs/ENB/Commissioners of Education & Training

R40   *We recommend that action is taken to safeguard money available under Working Paper 10 arrangements.*

Lead action by   NHSME

R41   *We recommend that new training initiatives aimed at developing clinical supervision skills in senior clinical nurses are devised. We also recommend that newly qualified nurses and nursing students receive preparation in what to expect from clinical supervision.*

Lead action by   NHSME/ENB/Commissioners and Providers of Education & Training

R42   *We recommend that the United Kingdom Central Council for Nursing, Midwifery and Health Visiting considers the accreditation of appropriate prior learning for entrants to pre-registration programmes.*

Lead action by   UKCC

Written evidence

Community Health Councils

Association of Community Health Councils England & Wales

Blackpool, Wyre & Flyde, Community Health Council

Crewe Community Health Council

Darlington Community Health Council

East Berkshire Community Health Council

Harrow Community Health Council

Kingston & Esher Community Health Council

North Lincolnshire Community Health Council

North Allerton District Community Health Council

Norwich District Community Health Council

South Cumbria Community Health Council

South Tyneside Community Health Council

Worthing Community Health Council

Colleges & Universities

Argyll & Clyde College of Nursing & Midwifery

Bolton & Salford College of Midwifery

Epsom & Kingston College of Nursing & Midwifery

Newcastle & Northumbria College of Health Studies

SHSA, Rampton Hospital

Sir Gordon Roberts College of Nursing & Midwifery Northampton

Tayside College of Nursing & Midwifery

The Norfolk College of Nursing & Midwifery

The Suffolk & Gt. Yarmouth College of Nursing & Midwifery

University of Greenwich

Family Health Services Authorities/ GP Practices

General Practice Group, Ryde I.O.W.

Berkshire Family Health Service Authority

Cumbria Family Health Services Authority

Devon Family Health Services Authority

Humberside Family Health Services Authority

Kensington & Chelsea & Westminster FHSA

Liverpool Family Health Service Authority

New Court Surgery Wootton Bassett Wilts

North Yorkshire Family Health Services Authority

Nottinghamshire Family Health Service Authority

Salford Family Health Service Authority

Staffordshire Family Health Service Authority

Surrey Family Health Service Authority

Wiltshire Family Health Services Authority

Wirral Family Health Services Authority

Health Authorities

Barking Haverwood & Brentwood Health Authority

Blackpool, Wyre & Flyde Health Authority

Cambridge Health Authority

Cambridge Health Authority Community Health Services Unit

Cambridge Health Authority
Mental Health Services

Canterbury & Thanet Health Authority

Coventry Health Authority

Dorset Health Commission Health Authority

Gloucester Health Authority

Herefordshire Health Authority

Leeds Health Authority

North Bedfordshire Health Authority

North Derbyshire Health Authority

North East Warwickshire Health Authority

North Tyne Health

Northumberland Health Authority

North Western Regional Health Authority

Nottingham Health Authority/
Rushcliffe Mental Health Team

Redbridge Health Authority

Shropshire Health Authority

South East Kent Health Authority

South Tyneside Health Authority

South West Durham Mental Health

Southampton Community Health Services

St. Helen's & Knowsley Health Authority

Tower Hamlets Health Authority

Trafford Health Authority

Wandsworth Health Authority

Wessex Regional Health Authority

Wycombe Health Authority

NHS Trusts

Combined Healthcare Bucknall Hospital

Exeter Community Health Service Trust

Frenchay Healthcare Trust

Newcastle Mental Health NHS Trust

Nottingham City Hospital NHS Trust

Premier Health NHS Trust, Walsall

Ravensbourne NHS Trust

Southmead Health Services Trust

Thameslink Healthcare Services Trust

United Bristol Healthcare Trust

West Dorset Mental Health Service Trust

Western Area Health Trust, Avon

Professional Organisations

Association of Nurses in Substance Abuse
(ANSA)

British Association of Social Workers

British Medical Association

Community Psychiatric Nurses Association
(CPNA)

Federation of MH Nursing Organisations

Royal College of General Practitioners

Royal College of Midwives Trust

Royal College of Nursing

Royal College of Psychiatrists

Standing Advisory Group for CPN Education

The British Psychological Society

Health Service Unions

Confederation of Health Service Employees

Social Services & Local Authorities

Berkshire County Council

Berkshire Service Provision & Management Support Services (East)

Brent Social Services Department

Buckingham County Council

Charing Cross Hospital Department of Social Work

Cumbria Social Services

Hertfordshire County Council

Knowsley Metropolitan Borough Council

Sandwell Metropolitan Borough Council

Shropshire County Council

Solihull Metropolitan Borough Council

Suffolk County Council

Wigan Metropolitan Borough Council

Wiltshire County Council

Wirral Social Services Department

Statutory Bodies

English National Board (ENB)

Voluntary Agencies

Family Welfare Association

National Association for Mental Health

Patient's Association London

Richmond Fellowship for Community Mental Health

Individuals

Adshead S P	Lees G A
Argyle N	Lee S
Armitage P	Lewis E
Barker S C	Lindow V
Bull A	Mahood N
Burchardt N	Miller A L
Campling Ms	Miller R
Connolly J	Moliver A
Corcos C D	Mycroft P L
Coulson A	Nullatamby S
Cull A P	O'Shea F
Daly M	Owen M
Day M	Parker A
Dudley M	Pidd G
Fischer M D	Reilly M M
Forster J	Sage G C
Furly R	Samociuk G A
Glenholmes K	Sheehy B
Griffin S	Smaje J
Gutt R H	Smith S
Hadlington D	Sutherland C
Howarth S J	Taylor E
Ingram O	Waine W
James A C	Walker P
Jenkins G	Weir A
Johnson T B	Welsh T D
Layford L	White E

Consultative conferences

1 Bristol

16 February 1993

Region	Delegates
South Western	19
West Midlands	12
Oxford	15
Wessex	19
Others	9
Total	73

2 London

18 February 1993

Region	Delegates
South West Thames	19
North West Thames	14
South East Thames	21
North East Thames	19
East Anglia	19
Others	13
Total	105

3 Harrogate

1 March 1993

Region	Delegates
North Western	21
Trent	16
Northern	20
Yorkshire	21
Mersey	10
Others	12
Total	100

Oral evidence

Professional Organisations

Association of Nurses in Substance Abuse (ANSA)

British Psychological Society

Community Psychiatric Association

Psychiatric Nurses Association

Royal College of General Practitioners

Health Service Unions

Confederation of Health Service Employees (COHSE)

Consumer Groups

Black Mental Health Association

National Schizophrenia Fellowship

The Patients Association

United Kingdom Advocacy Network (UKAN)

Individuals

Dr. Paul Armitage

*Special Hospitals and
Regional Secure Units*

Mr F. Powell

Mr H. Field

Mr P. Tarbuck

Ms G. Conley

Mr T. Hillis

Mr N. Maguire

North Manchester Community Team

Mr M. Greenwood

Mr M. Sly

Mr T. Ryan

Mr M. O'Flaherty

Visits to
clinical services

Newcastle Mental Health NHS Trust

Kings Lynn & Wisbech Hospitals NHS Trust

Camden & Islington Community
Health NHS Trust

Plymouth Community Health Services
NHS Trust

Derriford Hospital,
Plymouth Health Authority

Bradford Community Health NHS Trust

Entries and re-entries to Mental Health Nursing 1981-1993

Students

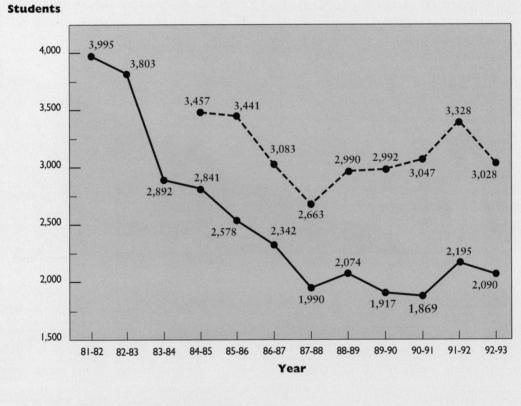

Source: English National Board

Nursing skills

Assessment

Self awareness

Awareness of one's own:

- values, attitudes, prejudices, beliefs, assumptions, feelings and countertransference and the management of these

- personal motives and needs and the extent to which these are being met

- competence, skills and limitations

- body language, including touch and gaze speech and other variables

- degree of attention to others

- genuineness and investment of self

  and how all the above might have an effect on others.

The intentional and conscious use of self.

Observing

- body language, voice, speech and physical state, in different settings

- the behaviour of the individual in relation to others including proximity and relative position

- how others react to the individual

- interaction with significant others.

Data collection

Awareness of sources of data – individual, family and significant others including other professionals.

Awareness and recognition of the factors which may distort data collection – emotional, cultural, environmental, language, transference/counter-transference, individual interpretations.

Awareness of range of available observations related to activities of daily living.

Determining the relevance and validity of data.

Awareness of the policies and procedures of the organisations in relation to the patients.

Arranging data in a logical way.

Interviewing

Formulating a strategy for the interview taking account of the uniqueness of the individual: age, sex, culture, race, class, religion, language style, personality, intelligence, previous observations and including the opening and closing of the interview. Choosing a time, arranging the environment, and duration of the interview with sensitivity to individual's needs/expectations. Agreeing a contract. Informing about self, the purpose of the interview and the limits of confidentiality.

Establishing rapport: reassuring the individual that no subject or language is taboo, and of the right of reticence.

Listening and attending.

Interpreting verbal and non-verbal communications.

Questioning about thought, feelings, expectations.

Drawing out by reflecting, paraphrasing, echoing, building and prompting.

Checking the precision and clarity of communication.

Ensuring the individual's need for self-expression is fulfilled.

Responding. Being flexible, intuitive, modifying and adapting the strategy and tactics, to the individual's needs, responses, wishes.

Being receptive and accepting; the non-judgemental approach.

Identifying needs and diagnosing problems

Awareness of factors which influence needs.

Classifying needs in terms of the individual's uniqueness.

Establishing priorities of need.

Appreciating the needs of the organisation.

Considering the needs of the individual against the value judgements of society.

Identifying the level of independency/dependency.

Assessing motivation, the degree of co-operation and constraints.

Making judgements based on all available data.

Identifying main and subsidiary problems.

Recognising issues amenable to nursing intervention and identifying those which need to be referred to others.

Setting priorities, ranking and ordering of nursing care needs.

Recording and disseminating information

Organising, documenting, charting, processing and assembling information.

Ensuring accuracy and compliance with legal requirements.

Compiling a nursing history. Ensuring confidentiality.

Ensuring that all relevant parties get comprehensive information without undue delay.

Planning

Identifying solutions

Reviewing, examining data systematically, taking account of all aspects, including relevant research.

Choosing approaches to problem solving.

Using problem solving skills to generate creative solutions.

Setting goals

Setting short-term and long-term objectives of nursing care, taking account of the policies of the organisation.

Formulating plans

Devising a strategy within the constraints of the organisation and taking account of ethical and legal implications.

Conceiving the plan of care.

Assessing the probability of success and failure taking account of potential risks and hazards.

Making decisions: logical and/or intuitive.

Assessing the reliability of decisions.

Setting the criteria of evaluation for measuring the achievement of objectives.

Ensuring adherence to the organisation's policies.

Communicating

Explaining clearly the purposes of the plan to the individual and the team.

Conducting a nursing care conference.

Gaining the trust of the individual, relatives, and friends, and promoting effective communication with colleagues and other groups.

Resolving difficulties in communications.

Negotiating the care plan with the individual and the care team.

Liaising with non-nursing personnel.

Sharing ideas. Discussing nursing diagnoses, solutions to problems with the individual and the team.

Producing the plan

Writing a clearly expressed, unique nursing care plan which can be understood by all grades of the multi-disciplinary team.

Preparing for review meetings. Preparing information for others.

Implementation

Planned intervention

Focusing on the needs of the individual when instituting purposeful, deliberate intervention.

Initiating action and contributing nursing expertise in team situations.

Maintaining a clear view of the intended goals whilst implementing care.

Understanding the effects of nursing care on the individual and the group.

Recognising the effects of the setting on the behaviour of the individual and the group.

Modifying objectives in the light of further information.

Ensuring a safe environment.

Motivating

Developing rapport. Displaying belief in the intrinsic worth of the individual.

Presenting stimuli to arouse interest – using positive incentives, persuasion, suggestion, appropriate rewards.

Fostering group identity and solidarity.

Teaching

Identifying and agreeing learning needs.

Creating learning opportunities.

Facilitating self-assessment.

Assisting others towards self-direction; independent thought, goal setting and action.

Offering examples of appropriate behaviour.

Acting as a model of independent, mature behaviour.

Encouraging others to challenge, explore, question.

Providing feedback.

Assisting the individual to modify inappropriate behaviour.

Using role-play.

Assisting in the transfer of learning.

The teaching of principles that promote mental health.

Assisting the individual and family to recognise factors that may precipitate mental illness and to take preventative action.

Evaluating the effectiveness of teaching.

Managing

Managing self in response to a rapidly changing set of stimuli.

Managing one's own anxieties and handling conflict, confrontation and criticism from individuals and groups.

Co-ordinating the activities of a group, monitoring, maintaining impetus, using group skills and group techniques.

Maintaining a positive attitude.

Sensitivity to care environment.

Accommodating plans made by staff in other disciplines.

Meeting personal care needs

Providing a safe therapeutic environment.

Maintaining optimum physical state.

Assisting the individual to breathe.

Assisting individuals with eating, drinking.

Promoting continence, managing incontinence.

Providing for work, play and physical exercise.

Creating an environment conductive to rest, sleep.

Taking and recording body temperature, pulse, respiration, blood pressure.

Helping in the maintenance of personal cleanliness and hygiene, bathing and washing.

Maintenance of privacy, dignity and individuality; the use of personal clothing.

Enabling individuals to express personal identity and sexuality.

Promotion of independence.

Assisting the individual in the practice of religious beliefs.

Preparing patients for examinations, therapies.

Administering drugs.

Carrying out practical procedures related to the above, in line with agreed local policies.

Dealing with accidents and emergencies.

Organisation

Utilising total resources.

Exercising appropriate leadership.

Introducing new staff to the setting.

Motivating the team to achieve objectives.

Controlling and co-ordinating the nursing team plans.

Effective organisation of the environment.

Helping others to identity and meet their own learning needs.

Teaching and demonstrating where appropriate.

Effective deployment of nursing staff.

Evaluation

Defining results

Identifying methods of evaluation.

Stating criteria for evaluation clearly.

Obtaining feedback

Seeking feedback from and the impressions of others; whether observers, participants, patients or otherwise; about what was said and done; about how it was said and done; with their views on the effectiveness of oneself and the plan and the performance of the team.

Discriminating between what is valid and invalid, in this feedback.

Assessing results

Assessing the validity and reliability of data of the evaluation.

Assessing objectivity and subjectivity related to the data.

Analysing the data.

Synthesising into a whole.

Summarising the results achieved.

Assessing progress or the lack of progress made.

Identifying process changes required

Using the results of evaluation to reconsider nursing care plans.

Setting new objectives as a result of the evaluation.

Creating opportunities

Setting up and using support systems to make evaluations possible.

Identifying realistic short and long-term goals for change.

Identifying activities and programmes, which will achieve goals, including learning activities, courses, group activities, counselling, and/or personal growth work; peer support and mutual aid.

Reviewing overall performance

Reflecting on and reviewing one's interviews and interactions.

Identifying all the critical elements in the complex process of those interactions.

Reviewing with the team the results achieved.

Managing success/failure in achieving goals

Identifying what was effective and ineffective within the constraints.

Identifying one's own contribution to success and failure.

Taking pleasure in one's own skills and successes.

Accepting failure and one's own human fallibility.

Identifying ways to confirm one's own strengths.

Identifying, with help from others, what in one's own personality and experience may limit one's effectiveness.

Identifying learning activities to improve skills, personal and professional development.

Recording and communicating

Documenting the progress achieved against criteria.

Reporting objectively to the care team.

Discussing the data with the individual.

Carrying out a nursing audit – conducting a peer review.

Using a variety of methods of recording data.

Use of rating scales where appropriate.

Source: English National Board

References

(1) Psychiatric Nursing Today and Tomorrow: Standing Mental Health & Standing Nursing Advisory Committees (1968); Ministry of Health – Central Health Services Council

(2) Secretary of State speech to the RCN Congress, 27th April 1992

(3) Position Paper on Community Psychiatric Nursing. Confidential Report to the Department of Health (1992); Brooker C. (Unpublished)

(4) Position Paper on In-Patient Psychiatric Nursing. Confidential report to the Department of Health (1992); Ferguson K, (Unpublished)

(5) The Future of Nursing by the year 2000: A Delphi Study 1992; White E; University of Manchester Department of Nursing Studies

(6) National Health Service and Community Care Act (1990); London HMSO

(7) The Children Act (1989); London HMSO

(8) The Patients Charter, (El(91)128) London: Department of Health (1991)

(9) The Health of the Nation, A Strategy for Health in England; London: HMSO (1991) (Cm; 1674)

(10) Project 2000: A New Preparation for Practice; UKCC for Nursing, Midwives and Health Visiting (1986)

(11) Experiencing Psychiatry; Users views of services. Eds. Rogers A, Pilgrim D, Lacey R; Pub MIND/Macmillan (1991)

(12) Stress on Women Campaign Pack; National Association for Mental Health (MIND) (1992)

(13) Women's Experience Campaign Pack; National Association for Mental Health (MIND) (1992)

(14) Race & Culture in Psychiatry (1988), Fernando S: Tavistock, Rutledge

(15) White Skins White Masks: Mental Illness & the Irish in Britain: Greenslade L; Institute of Irish Studies, University of Liverpool; Paper presented to the British Sociological Association Annual Conference 25th March 1991

(16) Access to Health Care for people from black and ethnic minorities; edited by Bahl V, Hopkins A; Royal College of Physicians; London, Cathedral Print Services Ltd

(17) The Third Quinquennial National Survey of Community Psychiatric Nursing; White E (1990); University of Manchester Nursing Department

(18) English National Board News (1990), J Wilson-Barnet; Nursing standard 21 (4) 10

(19) Mental Illness – What Does it Mean? Health of the Nation; July 1993 Department of Health

(20) Keeping the Records Straight; A guide for Nurses Midwives and Health Visitors: NHSME Training Directorate (1993)

(21) A Vision for the Future; The Nursing, Midwifery and Health Visiting Contribution to Health and Health Care; Department of Health NHS Management Executive; April 1993

(22) Working For Patients, Department of Health London: HMSO,(1989) (CM:555)

(23) Working with Families: Caring for a Relative with Schizophrenia: The Evolving Role of the Psychiatric Nurse: Brooker C, Butterworth C, (1991): International Journal of Nursing Studies, Vol 28, No.2, P189-200

(24) Clinical Supervision and mentorship in Nursing, Butterworth A, Faugier J, (1992) London: Chapman & Hall

(25) Supervision: A Co-operative Exercise in Accountability, in Enabling and Ensuring; Proctor B, (1986)

(26) Department of Health and the Welsh Office Mental Health Act 1983; Code of Practice 1993; London HMSO

(27) The Mental Health Act 1983, London HMSO

(28) Care Programme Approach (CPA) For People with Mental Illness Referred to the Specialist Psychiatric Services; HC(90)2/LASSL(90)11

(29) Secretary of State for Health announces ten-point plan for developing successful and safe community care; Press Release; Department of Health; H93/908

(30) Survey of English Mental Illness Hospitals; Davidges M, Elias S, Jayes B, Wood K, Yates J: Mental Health Taskforce October 1993

(31) Mental Illness the Fundamental Facts; Dr. Dick Thompson, (1993); Pub: Mental Health Foundation

(32) Homeless Mentally Ill Initiative (HMII) Department of Health (1990)

(33) Psychological Responses to HIV, Koenig C (1993); Conference Paper presented to European Association of Nurses in AIDS Care; Budapest 8th – 12th September 1993

(34) Sexual Abuse of Women in Psychiatric Hospitals: Copperman J; Camberwell Study; London School of Economics (Unpublished MSC thesis)

(35) Childhood Sexual Experiences with Adults: reported by female Psychiatric patients, Palmer RL; Chaloner DA; Oppenheimer R; British Journal of Psychiatry (1992) 160 pp261-265

(36) Working with adult survivors of child sexual abuse, Campling P; British Medical Journal (1992) vol.305 pp 1375

(37) Health of the Nation – Key Area Handbook for Mental Illness, Jan 1993 Department of Health

(38) A Review of a Psychological Intervention for Depression in Elderly People; Hughes C, (1993)

(39) Review of Health and Social Services for Mentally Disordered Offenders and Others Requiring Similar Services (1992); London HMSO (Cm 2088)

(40) Legal Powers on the Care of Mentally Ill People in the Community; Report of an Internal Review; Department of Health (1993)

(41) Care Custody and Justice – The Way Ahead for the Prison Service in England and Wales; Home Office, London HMSO (1991)

(42) Research For Health; Peckham M; Department of Health (1993)

(43) Report of the Strategy for Research in Nursing, Midwifery and Health Visiting; Department of Health (1993)

(44) The Contribution of Research to the Understanding of Nursing: McFarlane J (1981); Journal of Adv. Nursing 6 pp 231-241

(45) Better Services for the Mentally Ill (1975); Department of Health

(46) Generalising Research in Mental Health Nursing: Butterworth T (1991); Int. Journal of Nursing Studies Vol.28 No3 P237-246

(47) Training Community Psychiatric Nurses to undertake psychosocial intervention: report of a pilot study; British Journal of Psychiatry 160 86-844; Brooker Tarrier Butterworth Goldberg (1992)

(48) The Taps Project. 13: Clinical and Social Outcomes of Long-stay Psychiatric Patients after 1 year in the community; Anderson J, Dayson D, Wills W et al (1993); British Journal of Psychiatry (1993) 162 (suppl 19), 45-56

(49) Evaluation of Community Psychiatric Nursing in General Practice -in- Community Psychiatric Nursing: Research perspective; Illing J, Denewater D, Rogerson T, 1990: Ed. Brooker C.: Chapman & Hall

(50) The Nurses Midwives and Health Visitors Act (1979), DHSS, London 1990

(51) Working For Patients: Education and Training; Working Paper 10: Department of Health; HMSO (1989)

(52) Post Registration Education and Practice (PREPP); UKCC (1993)

(53) Framework for higher award for continuing professional education for Nurses Midwives and Health Visitors; English National Board (1991)

(54) The Integration Project – a Care Sector Consortium project (1991)

(55) National Occupational Standards for Care (OSC) Care Sector Consortium (1992)

(56) Requirements of Entry to Pre-Registration Nursing and Midwifery Programmes using Vocational Qualifications; UKCC Registrar's letter 31/1992 (1992)

Printed in the United Kingdom for HMSO
Dd 297804   C50   3/94   65536   3400   278283   08/29295